Taking the rough
with the smooth

TAKING THE ROUGH WITH THE SMOOTH

Dietary Fibre and your Health – a new Medical Breakthrough

by
Andrew Stanway MB, MRCP

With a Foreword by
DENIS BURKITT,
MD, FRCS(ed), FRS, D.Sc.(Hon), FRCSI(Hon)
and recipes by Dr Susan Heaton

SOUVENIR PRESS

First published 1976 by Souvenir Press Ltd,
43 Great Russell Street London WC1B 3PA
and simultaneously in Canada by
The Carswell Company Ltd,
Ontario, Canada
Reprinted April 1976

ISBN 0 285 62227 7

Printed in Great Britain by
Fletcher & Son Ltd, Norwich

TO MY WIFE
without whose expert help
as both doctor and cook this book
would not have been possible

Contents

Acknowledgements 8
Preface 10
Foreword by Denis Burkitt, MD, FRCS(ed), FRS, DSC(hon), FRCSI(hon) 12

One: Feeding ourselves to death 15
1 Man at the crossroads 17
2 The dilemma of Western diseases 22
3 Something in our food? 38
4 What is fibre? 41
5 What have they done with our fibre? 51
6 The discovery of fibre 58

Two: Fibre and disease 71
7 Dental caries . . . the tooth, the tooth and nothing but 73
8 Obesity . . . killing off the fat of the land 84
9 Diabetes . . . sugar, the vice of all things nice 95
10 Gallstones . . . rocks for ages, made by me 102
11 Coronaries . . . the way to a man's heart 109
12 Bowel disease . . . the real pressures of the Western world 122
13 Bowel cancer . . . the growth of interest in fibre 147

Three: Living with a high-fibre diet 153
14 What should I eat? 155
15 High-Fibre Diets and slimming 174
16 High-Fibre Diets in everday life 177
17 Some delicious High-Fibre recipes 193

Four: Can it really all be true? 239
Selected Bibliography 245
Index 251

Acknowledgements

It's often said in medicine that one is only as good as one's colleagues. This was never truer than of the fibre story: as with any new advance, everyone is feeling his way and relying upon colleagues and friends to help modify his recently acquired knowledge.

So it has been with me. For two years I have been in frequent personal contact with the leading figures in dietary fibre research and consider it a privilege to have been so. Their unending help and enthusiasm for the subject has made my job of writing about this medical discovery not only possible but thoroughly enjoyable.

I am especially grateful to the following:
Mr D. P. Burkitt, Medical Research Council, London
Dr T. L. Cleave
Dr J. Cummings, Medical Research Council, London
Dr M. Eastwood, Edinburgh Royal Infirmary, Scotland
Dr K. Heaton, Bristol Royal Infirmary.
Mr N. S. Painter, Manor House Hospital, London
Dr L. Silverstone, The London Hospital Dental School, London
Dr D. Southgate, MRC Dunn Nutrition Laboratory, Cambridge
Dr H. Trowell
Dr A. R. P. Walker, Director, Human Biochemistry Research Unit, Johannesburg

I am also grateful to the librarians of King's College Hospital Medical School and the Royal Society of Medicine, who have all been helpful, and to the Allinson family who so kindly allowed me to quote from Dr Allinson's works.

Section 3 would have been impossible to write without the help of Dr Susan Heaton who, with seven years experience of high-fibre cooking behind her, was a tower of strength when it came to the practicalities of feeding a family on high-fibre foods. Her recipes have stood the test of time, are completely in keeping with an unrefined, high-fibre diet and what's more, they're delicious!

Preface

'Oh, no!', I can hear you say, 'not another book telling me what *not* to eat!' No need to despair – this is no book for the food faddist or 'health food nut' – it's more a way of looking at the food we eat with new eyes.

For far too long we've all been obsessed with food additives, cholesterol, fatty acids and a host of other dietary red herrings. Certainly, some food additives are harmful – very high levels of cholesterol are bad for the heart, and fatty acids damaging to our arteries – but we've never been able to tie the dietary loose ends together and make a sensible, cohesive picture which explains our modern diseases.

For most of this century dietary medicine has devoted itself to curing the deficiency diseases, but staring us right in the face has been the greatest dietary deficiency of all: a lack of dietary fibre.

The story of dietary fibre is the classic one of finding only what you look for. Everyone knows that oxygen in the air is essential for life; but how many realise that the inert four-fifths of the air composed of nitrogen is also important? We certainly don't use it as such, but if too much oxygen displaces some of the nitrogen we're in trouble and become ill.

So it is with the roughage in our food. Always considered to be a waste product and of no use to our bodies, we now find that many of our modern diseases are caused by eating *too much* of the nutrients in food and *not enough* of the roughage. So just as too much oxygen without its nitrogen can be hazardous, so also can too much food without its dietary fibre.

It's so simple it's hardly believable. Whoever would have thought that something so basic and so long ignored as the roughage in our food could fire the imagination of doctors and scientists the world over? With more than a thousand scientific papers now published on the subject, fibre deserves the attention of every thinking man and woman. This is a discovery we ignore at our peril.

Foreword by Denis P. Burkitt

MD, FRCS(ed), FRS, DSC(hon), FRCSI(hon)

Appreciation of the value of high-fibre diets is not a recent phenomenon, nor for that matter are controlled dietary trials. Probably the first to be described is recorded in the first chapter of the Old Testament book of Daniel. He and his Israelite companions had been taken prisoner to Babylon by King Nebuchadnezzar, and singled out to be trained for high office. When offered the rich food of the palace they asked for permission to continue eating the fibre-rich food to which they were accustomed (only vegetables). The King's steward believed this to be an inferior diet to the one he was offering, but yielded to persuasion and mounted a controlled clinical trial, the young Israelites being the co-operating volunteers and those on the palace diet, the controls. The high-fibre diet won the day, those consuming it appearing healthier than the controls after the specified period of time.

From those days, but particularly since the progressive removal of fibre from food, the value of dietary fibre has been stressed by occasional perceptive individuals from time to time. The message has, however, never really got through either to the medical profession or to the lay public. Partly to blame for this have been the writers whose enthusiasm has outstripped their knowledge and judgement, and unorthodox commercial enterprises whose interests have often lain more in financial gain than in conformity to tested truths regarding dietary requirements.

In recent years there has been a steady accumulation of well attested evidence, both epidemiological and experimental, indicating unequivocally that the fibre in plant foods is as essential for the maintenance of health as are the other components of diet. Fibre has without doubt been the most neglected aspect of human nutrition, though its importance has for long been appreciated by veterinary scientists. It has in fact been considered a contaminating impurity rather than a dietary requirement, hence the word 'refining', which implies the removal of impurities.

The medical profession throughout the world is becoming increasingly aware of these facts. But for the message to have its maximum impact, it must be successfully communicated to the man in the street.

The widespread practical application of this knowledge could confer immense benefits, not only in reducing the incidence of major health problems in western countries, but also in saving peoples in developing countries from following our faulty footsteps in matters of food. No one interested in health can afford to ignore the facts presented here.

The majority of books written for the general public which have endeavoured to relate diets to health, have tended not only grossly to overrate certain aspects of truth, but also to cloud the issues by ascribing blame to many dietary changes without adequately examining the evidence which they present in support of their claims. Facts have frequently been distorted to endorse the writers' often foregone conclusions.

Dr Andrew Stanway has avoided these pitfalls. He has acquired a deep and wide knowledge of his subject and his work bears the imprint of a mind concerned to sift evidence and apportion credit or blame in the light of reliable scientific knowledge. His particular thesis, the fibre story, is presented both in the context of its historical emergence and of its relative relevance in the whole nutrition field. Moreover, the story is told and the argument presented in the manner of unravelling a problem and assembling the clues which must appeal to minds familiar with the plots of detective stories.

Dr Stanway's simple explanations of physiological and bio-chemical processes lay the essential foundations on which he constructs rational and compelling arguments to appeal to the reader's intelligence. All too often, the appeal of health literature has been emotional rather than factual.

The ever-growing volume of medical and scientific literature on this all-important theme has needed the complement of a scholarly yet simple account to impart important factual information to the layman. This is what Dr Stanway has ably provided.

Section one
Feeding ourselves to death

I Man at the crossroads

The days of our years are three score years and ten; and if by reason of strength they be four score years, yet is their strength labour and sorrow.

Psalm 90, v. 10

Man first appeared on this planet millions of years ago, since when he has progressed and evolved from ape man to the highly developed intellectual creature he is today. Over the ages man's fellow animals have also progressed. Some, like the dinosaurs, have come and gone, while others like the horse are still with us but in a physically more developed form. Man has made his great strides forward because he has developed a highly sophisticated nervous system which in turn has provided him with great dexterity, powers of reason and intellect.

Over the last century, a tiny fraction of man's evolutionary scale, he has so altered his environment and that of the animals sharing his planet that he has destroyed on average one species of animal each year. Man the destroyer is a relatively new phenomenon, probably only a century old, but now he's learnt how to do it, he's doing it with a vengeance. Man as the super-dominant species has opened a new chapter in the history of the world and it looks like being a bad one – not least for man himself. He seems bent on following his fellow animals to extinction.

Many of us, though, aren't prepared to sit back and accept this fatalistically.

The search for ways of prolonging life or at least for ways of postponing the ageing process has occupied men's minds for centuries. Indeed, it was our inability to accept that the ills assailing us were inevitable that first led to our interest in Medicine as a discipline. But if people were fascinated by the causes of plagues, pneumonia and syphilis for example, they were doubly enchanted by the thought that somewhere there might be a secret to life itself. Alchemists through the ages have searched for 'elixirs of life' and the idea of prolonging life has been the subject of thousands of papers, reviews, books and symposia.

Man has always wanted to live longer, irrespective of adverse circumstances. Many writings from Ancient times bear this out.

As we've become more civilised, though, the concept of living longer has become even more attractive as we have improved the quality of life by better housing, health and nutrition.

In past centuries, war, famine and pestilence made sure that of those who survived the childhood infections, few survived adulthood and even fewer reached old age. 'A baby born at the time of the Emperor Augustus could only expect to live for 23 years,' according to a paper in the Medical Journal of Australia (1964). It goes on, 'There was almost certainly no gain during the Middle Ages, but life expectancy slowly increased during modern times and by 1850 had reached 40 years. By 1900 another upward move had brought it to 47 years. Today, in most Western countries, life expectancy at birth has reached the impressive figure of 70 years.'

The author then goes on to warn, 'Our smug satisfaction with this achievement, however, needs correction. While in the last half century medical science succeeded in pushing life expectancy at birth up by some 20 years, the life expectancy of a 65-year-old during the same period has risen by less than one year. To put it bluntly, while we have almost eradicated infectious illnesses of childhood and adulthood, we have not succeeded in preventing degenerative processes and malignant growth, the two most common diseases of middle life and old age.'

This sobering view is not an individually held or even extreme one. As long ago as the 17th century, Halley of 'Halley's Comet' fame created the first life tables. He found that the expectation of life for a 60-year-old in 1687 was 12·09 years. Yet two hundred years later a 60-year-old had 12·2 years on average to live and by 1950 this had risen only to 15·7. So 263 years after the first of these surveys a 60-year-old was living just three-and-a-half years longer! At 60 and 80 respectively the expectation of life according to Halley was 12 and five years: today, nearly three centuries later, the figures are, for South African Whites, 17 and six years; for Australians, 17 and six years, and for American Jews, 15 and five years.

The two biggest killers over this period, childhood infections and epidemics of infectious adult diseases, killed enormous numbers of people and so drastically altered overall life expectancy. Infant mortality in England and Wales fell from 150 per thousand live births in 1838–1901 to 17·5 in 1965. Even if further reductions in infant mortality were to be made today it's unlikely that they would make much difference to the life expectancy of adults.

Epidemics have now been almost eliminated in the West. The impact of this achievement on the death rate can be judged from the fact that in 1849 in England and Wales cholera killed 50,000; in 1871–2 smallpox killed 42,000; and 1873 saw the death of 30,000 from scarlet fever – all this in a population of only 17 million.

So having conquered the major killer diseases over the last century, it seems surprising that we don't have a greater life expectancy.

Burch, in an article in the *American Heart Journal* in 1972, provided evidence that 'people live no longer any more', and made an excellent case for much more research into the process of ageing. His Annotation was salutory indeed and showed that in the USA, the life expectation at birth increased greatly this century until about 1950 when the graph flattened out. He went on to point out that the graph may now actually be *falling*. So it looks as though the expectation of life at birth reached its maximum about 20 years ago in the USA and that since then life expectation at middle age has slightly improved at 60 and not at all at 70. For the Jewish population of the USA since 1940 there has been an undoubted decline in life expectancy.

Burch's figures show that the expectation of life at birth has remained steady not only for Whites but also for non-Whites

(71 years for Whites and 64 years for Blacks). This is surprising to most people who would have thought that as the Blacks improved their socio-economic status they would live as long as the Whites. Perhaps, Burch suggested, the non-Whites are 'programmed' to have a shorter life span than Whites; but he added that he thought this unlikely.

Dr Walker, Director of the Human Biochemistry Research Unit of the South African Medical Research Council, has studied Indians living in India and compared them with Indians whose forbears had emigrated to South Africa. According to a general health survey carried out on a population of 73,000 rural Indians in South India in 1951, of the major causes of death, the first ten were infectious. People of 50 years old or more had a 14·5 per cent chance of reaching 70. Walker compared this data with similar information about Johannesburg Indians living in comfortable urban surroundings. Here, the main causes of death were coronary heart disease, pneumonia, strokes, cancer and diabetes. Of those aged 50 and over, only 9 per cent reached 70.

These studies showed that at middle age the urban Indians in South Africa had a somewhat reduced life expectation compared with their supposedly worse-off relatives back home in India. Studies have now been carried out in other comparable population groups and they all seem to lead to an inescapable conclusion. *Living in towns reduces our life expectancy.*

This is not simply an academic problem. How many of us know people in their forties, or even thirties, who have died of coronary heart disease – a condition almost unknown in two-thirds of the world? Our Western way of life seems to be killing us off younger, and it's picking off the men first. Women, on average, live longer than men in the West by as much as seven years. At an International Symposium on the causes of heart attacks, one of the speakers said 'Looking at total deaths in this country (the USA) we find that in the age group of our autopsies – mostly middle aged and elderly people – for the past ten years or so men have been dying off faster than women, at a rate of just below 3:2. If we go on at the rate we are going now, we will have a population of women entirely.'

So the situation is clear. Having overcome the great childhood killers, the epidemics and hopefully the wartime losses, if we want to reverse the trend of earlier death and wholesale sacrifice of our middle-aged men, we have to find cures for the main killing diseases of adulthood.

Having said this, I certainly don't propose such an advance solely in order to populate the West with centenarians. What we must aim for is a slowing down and hopefully even a halting of the rate of increase of the numbers of those suffering from these diseases. People are, of course, still going to die, but hopefully later rather than sooner and not after the long invalidism that so often accompanies our Western diseases.

Coronary artery disease is now affecting people under 45 more than ever before – a terrible prospect both for the families involved and for society as a whole, especially when one remembers that these men who are dying in their prime are also marrying later and leaving younger children behind.

Up to now man's diseases have at least allowed him to reproduce before he died. What if they now crept up on him at a younger and younger age until he didn't get that chance? How would society have to be reorganised to cope with millions more women than men? What are the political implications of so unhealthy and ailing a Western world?

I don't think we can sit around waiting for answers to questions like these. We need them today.

2 The dilemma of Western disease

Strange as it may seem, a handful of diseases kills off the same proportion of people in all Western countries. Coronary artery disease (heart attacks) kills about a third, cancer a quarter and strokes one seventh of the population. But these figures are for all ages. If we look just at middle age, heart disease kills one man in three, which is three times as many as die from all forms of cancer. The burden of this ill health on society is gigantic and is increasing throughout the Western world. In Great Britain today one in 100 of the population is in hospital at any one time, and a much larger, unfathomable percentage is in less than perfect health. The personal suffering involved cannot be overestimated, and the number of work days lost to industry far outnumbers that lost through strikes.

Yet much of our current health problem is a relatively new one. It's a little-known fact that coronary artery disease wasn't a recognised cause of death in England so far as death registrations were concerned until the mid-1920s. Tooth decay and gum disease too were uncommon before the latter part of the last century, as were diverticular disease of the colon, appendicitis and many others. We can say this with some certainty because medical literature, which abounded in the last two or three centuries especially, would have reported cases of these diseases had they been common.

As far back as Hippocrates, physicians were noting disease patterns and postulating causes for common ailments. It's unjust to suppose that until the present century doctors were incapable of recording what they saw, even though we don't have to accept the conclusions that they drew. There's little doubt that because of man's fascination with his own body and its workings, early physicians were no less assiduous in their studies than we are today. Certainly, they didn't have our modern armoury of diagnostic equipment, but the diseases that have 'appeared' this century rarely need electron microscopes and sophisticated biochemical tests to prove their presence.

On the contrary, physicians through the ages probably spent more time in meticulous post mortem examinations than do doctors today, if only because there were so few other ways of learning about diseases. Over the centuries we find immaculate descriptions of diseases, some of which are impossible to improve upon even in the light of present medical knowledge.

In recent centuries famous physicians and surgeons such as Thomas Sydenham, Lord Lister and Sir William Osler didn't see many of the diseases that are so common today yet they could scarcely be called amateurs. Osler reported only five cases of angina pectoris (the pain which may be the prelude to a heart attack) in 8860 patients he saw in 1893. Only thirteen years later he was able to report 268 cases in detail and only the serious ones would reach him at a hospital department, suggesting that the condition had increased greatly in incidence. Osler, one of the world's greatest physicians, commented at the turn of the century that it would be a lucky medical student who would see a case of coronary heart disease during his training. Today's medical student could easily see five new cases a week!

True, many people died with the label 'cause unknown' in times gone by; but certainly in the last century diagnostic methods, even if they were undertaken after death, were good enough to pick up at least occasional cases of our modern diseases. They didn't, so the diseases simply weren't there, or they were very rare indeed.

To come up to date a little more. Diverticular disease of the colon, a condition in which little 'blow-outs' appear in the wall of the large bowel, was very rare until the 1920s. Critics of this assumption point out that we make the diagnosis by X-ray and that such techniques were very poorly developed before the 1920s. But the little pouches formed in this disease are easily visible at post mortem and would have been readily seen had they been nearly as common as they are today. They now effect the bowels of 60 per cent of 60-year-olds . . . rather difficult to miss! In addition diverticulitis, a complication of this disease in which one or more of the blow-outs become inflamed, was reported as a rarity in the medical literature until the mid-1920s. Today it is a common and easily recognisable condition.

It simply isn't possible to believe that dramatic diseases such as these were missed or put down to other causes. In the Middle Ages, perhaps, but not a century ago. So we come to the unassailable conclusion that certain of our Western diseases are new this century. Why should this be so and has the same change in disease pattern occurred the world over? The answer quite simply is 'no'.

In the middle of the last century people were dying from cholera, smallpox, measles, scarlet fever and tuberculosis. As medical knowledge advanced, the old ideas of poverty and stresses and strains as being the *causes* of these diseases were displaced by new ideas on bacteriology and biochemistry.

For years, tuberculosis and rickets, the former an infectious disease and the latter a condition due to a deficiency of Vitamin D, were thought to be caused by the strains of low-standard urban living. The discovery of the tubercle bacillus meant that we could use a specific therapy to destroy it. Once it was known that rickets was caused by a deficiency in the diet, the missing vitamin could be restored.

So two so-called 'mysterious' diseases have been largely banished from our society.

The other major killers of the nineteenth century have also been eradicated from the West. Leprosy, smallpox, typhoid, scurvy, polio, scarlet fever and diphtheria rarely kill today in the West, but as fast as we've eradicated these, other new and more obstinate diseases have stepped in to take their places. The irony is that we, in the sophisticated space-age of the 1970s, are still putting these new diseases down to the same old causes that our forefathers blamed their diseases on – the stresses and strains of urban living. We're just as wrong as they were.

It would be foolish to pretend that the average man in the West today isn't a lot healthier than his predecessors as little as 100 years ago, let alone in the Middle Ages. However, things were not always as rosy, even in the recent past. The health of the British nation hit what was probably an all-time low as a result of the Industrial Revolution, which moved millions of people from country to town. Drummond and Wilbraham in their book *The Englishman's Food* report that the average man at the turn of this century lived almost entirely on bread and tea. Rickets and malnutrition were rife, and were found to be real drawbacks when recruiting men for the Army. Sir William Taylor, Director General of the Army Medical Service, reported that the Inspector of Recruiting was having the greatest difficulty in obtaining enough men of satisfactory physique for service in the South African War! The rejections in some areas were as high as 60 per cent, and over the country as a whole were 40 per cent. The chief grounds for rejection were, bad teeth, heart affections (not coronary artery disease), poor sight or hearing, and deformities. The lack of men was so serious that in 1902 they were forced to lower their height requirements and accept men of five feet – the previous limit had been 5 feet 6 inches.

By these standards nutritional levels have greatly improved throughout the West; yet this very improvement has become a double-edged sword as we shall see.

Although we're healthier overall and our standard of living has improved immeasurably, we seem to be living no longer *because our new diseases are negating the benefits obtained by curing the infections of the past.* This picture though, is not to be found all over the world; and the place to start our search for a possible answer to our urbanised Western dilemma, is strangely enough, in the underdeveloped countries.

Believe it or not, nearly two thirds of the world's population still suffers from diseases which were killing us a hundred years ago in the West. Cholera, tuberculosis, typhoid, malaria, smallpox and accidents still kill the majority of people in Africa and Asia. So striking is the difference in disease patterns in developed and developing countries that it led Dr Hugh Trowell, a physician in Africa for 30 years, to write a book on the subject in 1960. He looked at the levels of non-infective diseases in

Africa, which at that time had a population of 100 million, and found some amazing things. Gallstones, inflammation of the gallbladder, coronary artery disease, angina, pulmonary embolus, dental decay, diverticular disease of the colon, piles, cancer of the colon, appendicitis, disseminated sclerosis, brain tumours, thyroid disease, diabetes, rheumatoid arthritis and obesity were all uncommon or never seen in Africans.

Now it so happens that many of these diseases are the new diseases that we've seen emerging in the West this century. It struck him as being rather strange that as these diseases were mostly not inherited and were certainly not 'infectious', that their incidence wasn't the same in Africans and Whites. There was also a marked difference in these diseases among Africans living in towns and those living in villages. It wasn't as if these differences in occurrence were so small that it required statistical analysis to prove – they were often hundreds of times less common or even never seen in Africa at all outside the big cities.

Critics will say that there simply aren't the diagnostic and other skills in Africa that there are in the West to ensure that these diseases are diagnosed. This simply is not so. Many hundreds of highly skilled British and American doctors have worked in Africa for thousands of cumulative man-years – many with excellent diagnostic and therapeutic facilities – and yet they have never seen there some of the diseases we are concerned with. After all, if a distinguished British surgeon reports having seen only a handful of cases of, for example, appendicitis in a population of a million people over a period of so many years, one really cannot contend that he doesn't know what he's looking for!

So here in Africa we have a disease model comparable to that in the West a century ago. Could we perhaps watch Africa and Asia for the next century and see if they too start to get our modern diseases?

It hasn't been necessary to wait that long because here we are in only 1975 and we've seen it happen before our very eyes.

As people in Africa, or indeed in any developing country,

move from their rural surroundings into towns, they take on our Western way of life and with it our Western diseases. This finding has been so dramatic and so often repeated wherever we look in the world, from the Eskimo to the American Indian, from the African to the European, that there can no longer be any doubt. *These new diseases have something to do with living in towns.*

Before we look at which of the many changes associated with urban life could be at the root of these new diseases it might be helpful to see how certain parameters of Westerners and of people in developing countries differ. It's possible that a study of things such as growth rate, body weight, blood pressure levels, and blood fat levels might lead to a better understanding of the marked differences in disease patterns.

The growth of children in primitive and underdeveloped countries is almost always slower than in the West. Increased prosperity and nutrition increases growth rate. But is this desirable? The food tables of the world have been calculated on our Western 'needs' and are centred around our ideas of what good nutrition entails. Are African children to be compared with children in Ohio or Hanover? Probably not, especially as we now know from work among animals that faster growth makes for earlier senescence. Two hundred years ago English children attained maximum height at about 25 years. Today the age is more like 16 years, and in rural Africans it is about 20 years. Does the slower growth rate of the African make for slower ageing? Dr Walker of the South African Medical Research Council thinks it does. 'It is of interest to note that, allowing for differences in population numbers, in South Africa there are at least 20 times more Bantu over 100 years old than Whites. Whilst the ages of many of the former are uncertain, there is no doubt that, proportionately far more Bantu than Whites do reach a greater age.' Could it be that our faster degeneration and ageing in the West is something to do with our accelerated maturation?

Body weight is another parameter that differs in the two populations we're discussing. Most primitive or simple rural people gain little or no weight after they reach adulthood. Once they go into the towns they put on weight quickly. It's a well-known fact that the average Western child or adult today weighs more than his counterpart a century ago. The average height of the English child has increased one inch per generation and the average weight by an even greater proportion. In fact obesity is now an enormous problem in the West, as we shall see in chapter eight. Young and middle-aged men now weigh 15 lb more on average than 30 years ago, and the average US white man and woman are 19 and 15 lb respectively heavier than their British counterparts. This gain in weight is now thought to be a major factor in the large increase in heart disease, so it cannot be taken lightly. Middle-age spread, so often taken for granted in the West, is unknown in rural primitive peoples and so can hardly be considered normal.

Overweight matters because if you're fat your chances of fatal heart disease are doubled. Your chances of getting diabetes are three-and-a-half times greater; of dying from kidney disease, two-and-a-half times greater, and you're more likely to have a stroke. Life Insurance tables show that if you are severely obese and forty years old, instead of living to 72 on average, you'll only reach 65!

Critics point to the starving millions in the developing world and remark that the reason they don't get obese is that they haven't enough food. This may very well be true for some areas but there are also whole communities that have food in abundance and still don't get obese. There is even evidence that certain African tribes take in very large amounts of food (in terms of calorie intake) and still don't get fat. Could it be that they are immune to getting fat? Unfortunately not, because when these very people start eating *our* foods they get fat very quickly just as we do.

Closely linked to overweight is high blood pressure. Some primitive rural communities show no rise in blood pressure with age, although we in the West accept such a rise as 'usual' if not 'normal'. With urbanisation blood pressure levels rise, and in some groups this rise is enormous. One investigation among Natal Africans between the ages of 45 and 64 showed that the proportion of the population with high blood pressure went up from 36 per cent to 59 per cent as they moved from village to town. Similar rises in blood pressure on urbanisation have been reported from places as different as Easter Island, New Zealand, India and Russia.

Blood pressure and its related disease, atherosclerosis, are now thought to be 'the most commonly encountered chronic diseases in US adults', according to one leading authority. Just as with obesity, you stand a much greater (one-and-a-half times) chance of dying prematurely with high blood pressure than if you have normal blood pressure. If all deaths from cancer could be prevented, it would increase the average life-span of 40-year-old men by slightly over two years. If even moderately high blood pressure were curable, we could get an extension of four years. Quite a thought.

These are just a few of the parameters of health that we take as normal in the West, but yet which cannot really be con-sidered normal by the standards of many people in the world. So what is it that happens to men as they go into towns and become westernised?

Lots of changes occur as we all know, but if we disallow those for which there is no evidence linking them with modern Western diseases (such as television, air travel, playing bingo and a host of other urban pursuits blamed by a tiny minority), we're left with five possibilities: (1) reduced physical activity (2) stress (3) cigarette smoking (4) pollution and (5) altered diet.

Physical activity

Many primitive peoples are extremely fit. They spend a lot of their time taking physical exercise and perform well, even though possibly undernourished and certainly suffering from long-standing infections, compared with westerners under the same circumstances. Walker arranged races between white and Bantu children and found the undernourished Bantu quite up to the standard of the whites. Other studies have shown that the 'maximal oxygen intake' (a very good test of physical work capacity) of poorly-nourished African boys at 4000 feet above sea level was as good as that of fit German and American boys in their home towns. This level of fitness does, however, fall as the African boys become urbanised.

To understand the importance of physical work in relation to disease, let's look at the historical picture. Until two centuries ago in the West 90 per cent of men worked on the land. Today, only 5 per cent of men in the USA do so, and many of these now perform with machinery what used to be done with their hands, and so are sitting down a lot of the time. In an editorial in the *American Heart Journal* in 1966, Passmore called the Americans 'gluttons for sedentary work. At a recent medical conference in New York during January, a visitor could not but wonder that the lecture hall was packed with people from 9 am to 6 pm six days of the week, yet, when walking in snow-covered Central Park before breakfast he was as lonely as on a Scottish moor.'

Studies from many parts of the world have confirmed that physical inactivity is linked to an increased risk of coronary artery disease, and some say by a factor of three-and-a-half times. Among least active smokers the differential was nine times that among the most physically active non-smokers.

This said, there's almost no evidence that increased activity *per se* is of any benefit to middle-aged people. The trouble with all the studies done so far is that they have looked at exercise as one phenomenon among others. We shall soon see that this is wrong. Surgeon Captain T. L. Cleave puts exercise into its proper perspective when he points out that lack of exercise cannot possibly be blamed for coronary or indeed any other modern disease. He continues 'a lack of exercise cannot remotely be compatible with human evolution, especially as (it) is never considered in association with natural desires in these matters. For with regard to exercise, evolved sensations tend always to keep physical exercise in any pastime to the agreeable minimum, in order to reduce wear and tear on the body in general and on the heart in particular. To advise someone, who wants to rest, to take exercise is as unnatural as to advise someone who wants to throw himself into the fight and get on in the world, to moderate his effort.' He then goes on to point out that hermits, who take little exercise, are notably long-lived and that caged zoo animals also live a very long time. These seem very sensible arguments and are difficult to disprove.

Exercise lack has become a fashionable target for medical and lay 'do-gooders' alike, but it is by no means the evil it has been made out to be. The only grain of sense in taking more exercise than you feel you need is in order to lose excess weight you've put on by eating the wrong foods (see chapter eight) and then you need to take so much of it that it's doubtful if you will ever do it. After all, it takes a climb up a fair-sized mountain to get rid of the energy taken in at a single slap-up dinner. A walk around the block with the dog is only a token!

Stress

One hundred and fifty years ago Wordsworth wrote 'The world is too much with us; late and soon, getting and spending, we lay waste our powers.' Only 50 years ago Muller, writing in the *Annals of Life Insurance Medicine*, wrote the following remarkable passage:

There can be no doubt that modern man wears himself out more rapidly than did his forebears. Competition is keener, work is more exacting and technical advances make increasing demands. There is little, alas, that we can do to change this state of affairs. The railway, the motor car, the aeroplane, the telegraph and telephone have contributed only in appearance to ease of living. This armed peace exerts slower but more continuous pressure than many a previous war.

The problem with discussing stress is that it's impossible to measure. True, some of the body's chemicals (especially adrenaline and noradrenaline) are raised in stressful situations, but the conditions that are considered stressful by one person may be thought restful by another. As is pointed out in chapter one, we are not the first to have suffered the stresses of urban-ised Western living. Our ancestors were dogged by poverty, famine, bad housing and constant ill health – can we say that they were *not* stressed by these? That would seem very un-likely. Rural Africans and Asians today have much the same pressures to cope with as did our ancestors. Just imagine the average Western family coping with chronic ill health, shortage of food and water, poor transport, little or no housing, high infant death rate, repeated pregnancies and so on. They'd be stressed all right!

But there are different sorts of stress and it's possible that they affect us differently. Herd stresses, suffered by society as a whole (such as war, famine and national disasters), may well have different psychological and physical effects from personal stress. But whatever the answer, it's quite unreasonable and also inaccurate to put our modern diseases simply down to stress. Certainly, there are stresses we have that primitive people don't, as Muller pointed out: the breakdown of the family structure, intense job competition, the pressure for educational prowess and the constant demands to readapt to new inventions all contribute to them. But it's impossible to say that these are any more stressful or likely to cause disease than any stresses a rural African has to suffer. Studies have been able to indicate that heart attacks, strokes and certain other Western diseases are caused in part by stress – but there's just as good a correlation between these diseases and, for instance, the number of television licenses sold: the graphs are almost exactly parallel. Yet who would suggest that TV licenses *cause* heart attacks?

This will, I realise, be a very hard pill for the average reader to swallow, but that's because he'll have thought of the rural African's life as one of unending bliss seated under a tree all day waiting for the relief agencies to bring him food. After discussions with doctors who have between them more than 100 man years experience of Africa, I can assure you that this is not so.

According to Captain Cleave 'The very mainspring of evolution has always consisted of the struggle for existence, where the killing of one organism by another represents stress in its starkest form. If we are adapted to anything in this world, we are certainly adapted to stress.'

Cigarette smoking

Many primitive communities don't smoke tobacco, but as they come into contact with Westerners they tend to take the habit up. This is undoubtedly an important health hazard on two fronts – heart disease and lung cancer.

Lung cancer is now the commonest cancer in Western men, and heart disease the commonest cause of non-cancer death, so it's certainly worth stopping smoking. Heavy smokers have a death rate two to three times greater than non-smokers, but on giving up the habit the risk is reduced over a long period to normal or $1\frac{1}{2}$ times normal.

But cigarette smoking clearly can't be the sole cause of any of our Western diseases because some people who have never smoked still die from lung cancer and lung disease, for instance. Smoking is only a predisposing factor in some of these diseases. It is probably causative in lung cancer, but as yet, there is no evidence that smoking is the primary cause of any of the other diseases we're discussing.

Pollution, television, jet travel etc

All these facets of modern urban life have been blamed by someone at one time or another yet there's little evidence that they cause any of the diseases we're discussing. Lead pollution causes all manner of ills from backward children to anaemias, and mercury poisoning too is undoubtedly dangerous. Yet pollution, including the long-term build up of DDT in our bodies from the foods we eat, doesn't seem to cause appendicitis, cancer of the colon, heart disease or the other special problems of the West. There may be an as yet unforeseen danger in something as simple as the exhaust fumes from motor cars, in addition to the known lead hazard, but extensive tests have so far proved this unlikely.

There will always be those who seriously consider that jet travel, television or the landing of men on the moon is the root of all our ills, but there is absolutely no proof that any of these things has any impact at all on any of the diseases we're discussing.

So last, but obviously not least, we come to food.

Food

This is worth serious consideration for one very simple reason: many of the diseases that are new, both to us in the West over the last 100 years and to primitive people moving from village to town, are diseases of the bowel, or are linked to such diseases. Even heart disease, seemingly a far cry from the bowel, is now thought by some to be associated with obesity. Studies of coronary heart disease in seven countries showed that it was not *necessarily* linked to obesity, and it's possible that the dangers have been overplayed, but until we know for certain it's probably safer to control obesity in any case because of its undoubted hazards for other parts of the body.

Because dietary changes, both over the last century in the West and as villagers move into towns in the developing countries, are so important, we must look at them in more detail.

3 Something in our food?

Dietetics, the study of food, is a very young branch of science and could scarcely have been called a science at all until the middle of the last century. Even the term 'diet' was used very loosely to include air, food, exercise, rest, sleep and so on until the early 1800s. That's not to say that man hasn't been interested in food for centuries. The Bible has references to foods and their values in certain illnesses and Hippocrates, Galen and Celsus, the three greatest of Ancient physicians, took up the subject with a vengeance. Hippocrates recommended that the diet be plentiful in winter and sparing in summer. He disapproved strongly of the new white breads and pointed out that the meat of wild animals was more easily digested than that of domesticated ones. Many of his theories though were empirical to say the least. Few were based on experimental data and he, along with the other great thinkers of the day, was very much bound to semi-metaphysical theories. With the writings of Galen, dietetics took a more modern turn. He wrote three books on the Faculties or Powers of Aliments, one of which contains 71 chapters on fruit and vegetables alone.

But it was in Medieval times that food was first linked to disease in a truly cause-and-effect way, when foods were divided into two kinds. The first brought about a 'good humour' and the others a 'bad humour'.

Foods producing a good humour were thought to generate good blood and included fresh bread and flesh of a lamb or kid. Bad humour was produced by bad bread and flesh of old beef and goats. Some vegetables were also held to produce evil humours and heavy foods were avoided because they gave rise to phlegm and black bile.

These ideas about food influencing the humours persisted

until the early 19th century, when chemistry, by then far more advanced than most dieticians would admit, started to make an impact on dietetics. Paris's *Treatise on Diet* published in 1839 was probably the first book to deal with food in what we would call a modern way. Chemistry, together with new work on physiology from Germany, began to impinge on dietetic thought and by the 1870s the relative values of different foods and their equivalents in heat and work had been well documented.

So almost within living memory the study of food has become a respectable science. But if the 19th century marked the beginning of our understanding of the qualities of foods, the 20th has been the time for our interest in food values and quantities. So having started this century fully aware that proteins, fats and carbohydrates were all necessary for health, we have spent most of the time since then examining the so-called 'accessory food substances'. These include the vitamins, the minerals and the trace elements.

Of all of these the discovery of the vitamins was probably the greatest single advance, because it showed conclusively that certain diseases, previously thought to be incurable, were easily remedied by adding simple things to the diet. But important as these accessory food factors undoubtedly are, their value mustn't be over-estimated. They are simply a fraction of a total diet which consists of many parts. Modern research has shown that all of these parts are equally important.

There is now known to be a host of diseases linked to deficiencies in various parts of our food. Lack of protein, fat, minerals or vitamins can produce diseases – some of them life-threatening. But even today we tend to divide the dietetic problems of the world into two camps. On the one hand there's the starving two-thirds of the world that seems to be suffering from deficiency diseases, and on the other hand the rich, Westernised third that, if anything, suffers from overnutrition. Just as there's a shortage of food in the developing countries so there is a parallel superabundance in the West, and the gap is getting wider.

This wouldn't be so tragic if by over-using food resources in the West we didn't prejudice those in the rest of the world. Unfortunately we do. We eat far more protein, fat and carbohydrate than we need, and by eating it in the form of meat from animals fed on expensive grain we deprive the starving millions of that grain. Grain is a more effective foodstuff when eaten in its natural state rather than converted into beef.

But as our knowledge of food has evolved over the years, so food itself has changed. These changes are not only in the amounts of food we eat but also in the kinds of food. Since the late 18th century sugar and starch consumption has changed profoundly. In 1770 the average Briton ate 500 g of flour a day; by 1970 this had fallen to 200 g. Between 1700 and 1850 sugar consumption was very low indeed, mainly because it was so expensive. The amount consumed has risen enormously since 1850 so as to make up the energy gap left by the lower consumption of flour and potatoes. We now consume in two weeks in Britain as much sugar as the Elizabethans got through in a year.

Fat consumption too has changed in the West. Before the Agricultural Revolution in Britain, fat consumption was low, probably about 25 g per day. In 1970 the average man ate 145 g per day and obtained 40 per cent of his calories from it. Much of this increased fat consumption has been due to the greater availability and popularity of milk and cheese which are also nutritious in other ways.

The overwhelming quantitative change, however, has been in the number of calories we consume. All Western nations have consistently increased their calorie intake this century, except during the periods of rationing in the two World Wars. This has occurred because of a greater consumption of carbohydrate and fat. (Carbohydrate provides four calories/gramme and fat provides nine calories/gramme of energy.) We shall see the price we are paying for this overconsumption in the chapter on obesity (see chapter eight).

Before we can understand how food changes might be responsible for some of the new diseases, we need to see how the food of rural people moving into towns has changed too.

Whilst any reader will know only too well what we eat in the

West, he may not know the kinds of foods that the other two-thirds of the world lives on. Obviously, we're discussing peoples as different as the American Indians, the Maoris, the Africans and the Chinese, so it's difficult to generalise. But overall they eat more whole or naturally occurring foods, mostly in the form of vegetables and grain, than we do. True, the Eskimo eats largely meat and fat and the Masai milk and meat, but predominently carnivorous human beings such as these are rare indeed. Primitive man and the higher apes were plant eaters.

Over the years, however, man has cultivated grasses for their seed (grain), and Western man has perfected agricultural techniques capable of feeding large numbers of people, many of whom live a long way from the source of their food.

Rural Africans and Asians today live very much as our ancestors did in the West. They are peasant agriculturalists growing, processing and eating their own food. Where they do grow grain they grind the seed between stones, so using all of it, including the outer coat or bran. In many rural areas starch from cereals gives the people 70–80 per cent of their calories. They eat very little fat and only moderate amounts of protein. If food is plentiful the adults do well, but if not children are the first to suffer and get diseases of malnutrition such as kwashiorkor.

As rural people become westernised their diets change to become more like ours. One of the first things to be added is sugar which is a good source of calories and stores well. As the people become richer they consume more fat and animal protein until eventually, when they live alongside Westerners in towns, they take on their diet completely. In their desire to benefit from the advantages of urban living (sanitation, water supplies, transport, housing and so on) rural people quite naturally want more sophisticated foods too. These are, almost without exception, more refined and processed than the natural foods they have been used to – and for a very basic reason.

For as long as a man is tied to producing the food he and his family need, he has to live near the source of that food. In a rural, mainly agrarian society, people produce enough food for themselves and their families. With the growth of towns most people live a long way from the source of food production and so have to rely on farmers, who produce food in large enough quantities to satisfy the demands of these urban populations. In order to supply enough food to a community throughout the year, this food must be storable. This presents a problem because most foods don't keep very well for long periods. The answer then is to process them in such a way as to prolong their life, prevent wastage and ensure continuity of supplies.

As grain was the staple source of energy in the West until this century, and indeed still is in the majority of rural communities in Africa and Asia, let's take it as an example and see what happens when we process it.

A grain of wheat or rice consists of several parts. Its bulk is the endosperm which, when milled, gives flour (starch). A smaller part is formed by the germ which contains protein, fat and mineral salts. The outermost layers of the grain contain the bran. Since it was first realised that stored wheat went bad because the fat contained in the germ became rancid, efforts have been made to remove the germ and so to make flour storable for long periods. We'll go into more detail in another chapter as to how this was achieved, but suffice it to say that by grinding up the grain between rollers in a flour mill not only is the germ removed but so also is the bran. Both germ and bran are sieved off to leave white flour. The removal of the germ was thought to be of little importance because we could so easily make up for its small protein and mineral content by eating other foods rich in these substances. Nobody thought that the loss of bran, the outer husk of roughage, was of any importance – until recently, that is, when it was realised that although our intake of protein, carbohydrates and fats has risen considerably over the last 100 years in the West, our intake of bran and of roughage in all forms has fallen dramatically. In fact, if the consumption of the major foodstuffs has risen two- or three-fold, our intake of dietary fibre has fallen by a factor of almost ten.

So while nutritionists and the food processing industry have been obsessed by food values and the numbers of calories produced per unit of food, something even more important has been slowly disappearing from our western food. The fascinating fact is that this tenfold fall in the dietary fibre in our food has taken 100 years to occur in the West, yet comparable changes in food fibre have been telescoped into a mere decade in Africa and other developing countries as the people become urbanised.

Of all the changes that occur as people leave their villages and go into towns the greatest seems to be that in their food. And probably the greatest single change in food is the reduction in dietary fibre or roughage. Could it be that the emergence of our new diseases in the West, and their appearance in the town-dwellers of Africa and Asia, are both caused by the same thing – a fall in the roughage or dietary fibre content of our food?

4 What is fibre?

Strangely enough, although dietary fibre is now a well recognised and much researched medical concept, no one really knows how to define it.

The idea that fibre or roughage was important in food came originally not from doctors but from vets and animal nutritionists. Ruminant animals, with their several stomachs (the rumen) and special intestinal bacteria, eat more fibre than man has ever done. Animal nutritionists obviously wanted to know what the leaves and shoots these animals were eating did for them in terms of food value. So most of our early knowledge of fibre came from scientists like these.

This sort of research has been going on for as long as 70–80 years, and there is a massive body of data on all sorts of roughage and how it affects animals. But for all this, very few people have actually used any of these findings when thinking about man, because they reasoned that as man was not a herbivore, he couldn't use plant roughage as food. And, because man didn't have a rumen (like a cow for instance), they argued that however much fibre he ate, he couldn't 'use' it – so why bother about it at all?

We now think that this policy was a mistake, because man is in fact an omnivore. Indeed, our ancient ancestors ate plant foods almost exclusively, as do the higher apes today, so our bowels must at some time have been able to cope with fibre-rich diets.

But what exactly is fibre?

Dietary fibre consists of the walls of plant cells. The walls of animal cells are of no concern to us here because we digest them along with the rest of the meat; but plant fibre is a very different substance.

All plants are made up of cells, just as animals are. Many animals can be as large as they are only because the great mass of their cells is held on to a strong support, the skeleton. Plants don't have skeletons as such, but they make up for the lack because each cell or collection or cells has its own exterior 'skeleton'. The plant cell-wall is in fact outside the cell proper. This strengthening material, the scaffolding that makes plants rigid and strong, is fibre. Many plant cell-walls, and indeed their contents, consist largely of fibre. But even among plant cells some are more specialised for supportive strength than others. Some plant fibres are very delicate (just cut through a tomato and see the semi-liquid inside) while others are extremely strong. But the skeleton of the giant 200-feet-high Canadian Redwood tree, and that of the tomato with its delicate lattice-work, are both made of the same thing – fibre.

Plant fibre is an extremely important commodity in everyday life. Many useful products, from timber, paper, cotton garments to foods for domestic animals, are made of it. We've thus learnt how to harness the valuable properties of fibre in many areas: yet are only just beginning to work out its importance in our own food.

Considering also that fibre is such a valuable commodity, we waste an enormous amount of it. It's been estimated that a quarter of all the trees ever grown is lost completely because their fibre is destroyed by conversion into paper and timber. New growth of trees cannot keep up with our insatiable demand for these commodities, so we are slowly building up a net fibre deficit. Millions of tons of fibre are also removed from foods during their refining, and much of this is either re-used badly or even thrown away altogether. With our modern interest in conservation, we certainly ought to be more concerned about this wastage of plant resources, which are every bit as important as oil and coal.

But which of all the naturally occurring fibres might be of value to us as food? To answer this we need to take a look at fibre in more detail.

The dietary fibre of plants is made up of a family of substances called the polysaccharides. These are linked chains of sugars bound together in various ways to give fibres of different lengths and properties. Here, I must demolish the myth that fibre is necessarily 'fibrous'. Certainly, the stringy parts of celery and green beans are fibrous but the soft centre of a tomato or a banana similarly contain fibre.

Dietary fibre is a broad term which covers all the plant scaffolding substances. In fact, fibre has been compared with the vitamins, so many and varied are the properties of each individual type. Some fibre is actually very 'smooth' and doesn't feel at all how you would expect 'roughage' to feel. Bran, for instance, is very smooth to the touch and yet is just as much fibre as is a piece of mahogany. Other fibres are so delicate and minute that you'd have difficulty in seeing them without a high-powered microscope.

Perhaps the best known member of the fibre family is cellulose. This is a strong substance that keeps plants rigid. A plant is erect because of its fibre content and the turgid nature of its cells. Cotton is almost pure cellulose. At one time, not long ago, scientists thought that fibre *was* cellulose but, as we're beginning to learn, this is far from the case. Pectin, the second member of the fibre family, is well known to jam makers and forms a sort of jelly when water is added. Its sticky, adhesive properties make it useful not only to the jam maker but also to the plants from which it comes. Apples and citrus fruits are especially rich in pectin.

Substances called hemicelluloses give plants their flexibility because of their 'plastic' properties, and lignins added to cellulose give the fibres of wood their strength. Lignin makes up about 12 per cent of the dry weight of an annual plant, for instance.

There are many more complicated polysaccharides in the fibre family, and new ones are being discovered all the time; but for the purposes of this book we'll stay with these four: cellulose, pectin, hemicelluloses and lignins.

But even these four groups of substances are very different from each other, and we clearly can't talk about the fibre in trees and in a soft fleshy strawberry in quite the same terms nutritionally.

The term 'dietary fibre' was used loosely early this century when people were just beginning to understand which parts of our food we use nutritionally and which parts we don't. It was realised many decades ago that fibre or roughage was a carbohydrate made up of different polysaccharides arranged in such a way as to form very different substances. But because these fibrous forms of carbohydrate weren't digested they were called 'unavailable carbohydrates' as opposed to the 'available' ones we eat for food (bread, sugar, potatoes and so on). In fact, the measurement of the proportions of nutrients in our foods was primitive until very recently; and even today the food tables of the world estimate fat by direct measurement and protein by estimating the nitrogen content, then assume that what's left is all carbohydrate.

It's a fascinating fact that fibre itself may in practice make some foods which are normally completely absorbed by the bowel less likely to be absorbed. This is because the rigid, tough outer coating of fibre around the nutritious starch or protein in a plant cell somehow protects it from being broken down by the digestive juices. To what extent exactly fibre interferes with or controls the digestion and absorption of foods is still not known, but research is well under way.

So far, I've made it sound very simple. Unfortunately it isn't. Fibre differs from many other substances in that although it can be extracted from plants for analysis, this very extraction process alters it so much that it's difficult to know what we're dealing with. Arguments on this have been raging for years.

Plants, or the parts of plants we use as foods, obviously don't consist only of fibre. We cultivate cereals for their protein and carbohydrate; olives for their oil; oranges for their juice and so on. But food substances are contained within a latticework of fibre which gives the whole food a structure and texture.

A tomato or a cucumber is well over 95 per cent water, as is a strawberry, yet we like the succulent texture of these fruits. A seed out of its husk is almost all 'food' to us, yet we have to eat the fibre along with the food material – unless we process the seed in some way to extract the oil. Nutritionists over the centuries have tended to concentrate on the nourishing parts of foods and have assumed that all the rest were of little or no importance – except to animals.

As early as 1860 people were looking at fibre as a source of food for animals and trying to estimate how much nourishment it contained. These early researchers reasoned that if they dissolved out those parts of the plant generally accepted as being nutritious (by boiling with acids, alkalis and solvents) then the remainder would be the 'indigestible' fibre.

Sadly, these methods, although still used today, are pitifully inaccurate. Even with modern solvents and today's knowledge of chemistry we still don't know if we are really extracting all the nutrients and leaving only the fibre. The strong acids and alkalis used also probably affect the very nature of the fibre itself, so altering it completely from its natural state.

Food analysts officially define (crude) fibre as 'that portion of foods, or faeces, which remains after boiling with ten times its weight of sulphuric acid, filtering and boiling the residue with ten times its weight of alkali'. Such drastic treatment could scarcely be compared with the working of our digestive juices, so the definition may be of little value.

What we seem to have lost sight of is that man was originally a fruit and plant eater and later became a grain eater, and that for millions of years he has lived on a combination of fruit and grain. Somehow his bowels managed well enough, or he wouldn't have lived to tell the tale! Yet even today people say 'If we were meant to eat roughage we would have been given a stomach like a cow's.' Certainly our stomachs no longer perform this function of plant digestion; but the signs are that are colons do.

Recent research suggests that we *were* in fact supposed to eat plant fibre and that our bowels can use it – not as a real source of food any more, but for other equally important things. So what does fibre do and how does it do it?

Because we are talking about a family of substances, each with their own individual properties, it's difficult to generalise. But there is one outstanding thing that most fibres do. They absorb large amounts of water. If you put some pectin powder into a glass and add water, after a few minutes' gentle agitation the whole mass will have swollen to form a bulky semi-solid substance. Similarly, cotton wool, which is almost pure cellulose, swells enormously when soaked in water.

Different fibres have different water absorbing powers. Wheat bran – the tough outer coating of the wheat grain – is probably the best 'sweller' of all fibre foods. This is partly because it's dry to start with; but wet fibre such as that contained in carrots, lettuce, mango and celery also absorbs large amounts of water. Some plant materials on the other hand absorb very little water. A turnip is one such.

This water-absorbing property is important for our bowels, because it gives food the bulk the bowel needs to make food pass along it. Foods low in fibre pass very slowly through the bowel and may remain in the colon for several days. We now know that this bulking action of the fibre we eat also helps to prevent certain diseases of the large bowel.

The most important of these is diverticular disease (see chapter twelve). This common condition of the large bowel in which small 'blow-outs' form because of abnormal pressures developing in the bowel as small hard stools are passed along, can be prevented or alleviated by eating a diet rich in fibre. The only beneficial effect of this treatment, as far as we know, is that the fibre increases the bulk of the stool so giving the diseased colon a larger, softer motion to pass.

But along with the water that fibre absorbs go many of the body's valuable chemicals, like sodium and potassium, which are dissolved in it. The human colon as we shall see later is not the useless septic tank it was once thought to be. Complex and essential chemical reactions take place there which seem to need fibre to work properly. People who have had their colons removed because of disease can live without them, but if you have a colon then you need fibre in your food.

Not only does fibre retain water, so making the stools larger, softer and easier to pass, but the extra bulk has other effects too, mainly on bacteria in the bowels. Inside the bowels of man and other animals are many different sorts of bacteria. In animals with a rumen these bacteria are especially equipped to digest plant fibre, so enabling them to live entirely on plant foods, but most of the bowel bacteria in man don't digest fibre any longer. We can digest some components of fibre, like pectin and hemicelluloses, but by and large it's fair to say that we don't actually get food value out of the fibre in plants. We simply haven't got the right bacteria to do it.

Studies of bowel bacteria in man, however, have shown that different communities all over the world have different types of bacteria in their colons, and that there are many ways in which Western patterns of colonic bacteria are associated with particular diseases. Another function of fibre, then, would seem to be to alter the bacteria in the bowel, and thus to affect vulnerability to certain diseases. This happens in several distinct but interlinked ways.

Some bacteria actually get caught up in the 'swollen sponge' of fibre, so getting trapped right up against the fibre itself, which may alter the way in which they behave. There is also less time for bacteria to breed in faeces with a high fibre content, because they are moved through the bowel so quickly. But what is most important of all is the fact that the actual types of bacteria change as people go on to or indeed give up high fibre foods. The importance of this in cancer of the colon is discussed later (chapter thirteen).

One of the main effects of increasing the bulk of the stools is that any substances, be they useful or harmful, are diluted by the greater mass of stools. This seemingly unimportant side effect of fibre is turning out to be vital in the study of the drugs and chemicals we eat. Researchers in the USA have found that laboratory animals fed on refined diets become ill or even die if they're fed certain food colouring materials, or indeed large quantities of cyclamate (the chemical sweetener). If the same animals have fibre added to their diets in addition to these chemicals, they thrive. So somehow the fibre protects them. Could it actually be absorbing the noxious chemicals or their by-products in the colon? The answer seems to be a qualified 'yes'. This fascinating group of experiments indeed raises the diet of laboratory animals used for testing new drugs and food additives as an important question. Unless they're eating the same types of diet as we, the drug takers, can we accurately say that the drugs or chemicals will be safe in man? Probably not, because in the first place our low-fibre diets in the West produce firm, concentrated stools in which any harmful chemical will have maximum effect on the colon wall; and in the second the food passes so slowly through the bowel when we eat low-fibre diets that any poisonous substances have maximum time to get absorbed into the blood stream and exert any possible harm on the body. Both the body's natural chemicals and any chemicals and drugs we eat seem to be passed out in the stools in amounts directly proportional to the weight of the stool passed. So the greater the stool volume the more efficient the clearing of harmful chemicals from the bowel.

The third property of fibre is that it acts like a water softener, exchanging certain body chemicals for others in the food. Plant cells have a strong affinity for certain chemical elements, especially metallic ones. This binding power is essential for the growing plant because these chemicals are needed in microscopic amounts for the plant's normal metabolism. When we eat a plant, the fibre of which it is made doesn't suddenly lose the intrinsic chemical properties which have made it so valuable to the plant itself. Instead, these very important properties continue to act in the bowel. Just which of them act for the good and which may be harmful is not yet known, but if we accept that we've been eating nuts, fruits and berries for millions of years, the chances are very high that our bowels have harnessed these plant-cell properties to our advantage. Who knows, by *not* eating them, we may actually be losing substances we can get in no other way.

Some experts feel that too much fibre might mean that valuable body substances like iron, calcium and magnesium might be bound on to the fibre and so swept out in the faeces. This seems unlikely in the light of present knowledge. On the contrary, there's every reason to believe that fibre-rich foods will regulate the chemical composition of the stools in ways which are advantageous to us.

So what foods contain the valuable fibre?

All foods of plant origin have some fibre in them. Some of the richest sources of all are the leguminous seeds – beans, peas, lentils – and the cereals. These can have up to 81 g of fibre per 1000 Kcals of energy supplied. Leafy vegetables such as cabbages also have plenty of fibre, especially when related the number of calories they contain: cabbage for example gives 100 g per 1000 Kcals. Other examples for comparison are: apples 36 g; whole wheat 36 g; and banana 44 g per 1000 Kcals.

Compare this with the lowest end of the scale, where sugar (refined) and white flour (70 per cent extraction) have almost no fibre at all. Brown bread contains a little fibre and mustn't be confused with wholemeal bread. Rice, if it's white, also has very little fibre, yet if brown is a rich source.

Fats, sugar, milk, eggs, fish, meat and alcoholic drinks contain no dietary fibre at all.

Bread has been called the staff of life and when made with wholemeal flour can be one of the major sources of fibre in the diet.

Until the end of the eighteenth century most people in the Western world ate wholemeal bread. Indeed wholemeal bread was the staple diet of the majority of the population for centuries, and supplied most of the protein, starch, minerals and vitamins the people needed. The whole grain of wheat, rice or maize is a remarkably nourishing and almost complete food.

We know fairly accurately how much bread was eaten at the end of the eighteenth century: about 600 g per person per day (1 lb). This meant that people were getting about 30 g of dietary fibre a day from bread alone. Since then our intake of fibre from bread has fallen to about a quarter of what it was, and possibly even less. But have we made up this fibre loss elsewhere?

The answer is 'no'. We certainly eat more fresh fruit and vegetables than our ancestors a century ago, but recent evidence shows that the actual amount of fibre in these fruits and vegetables has fallen over the years.

It's a fascinating fact that even the humble carrot has changed its fibre content over the last 50 years. Seed manufacturers, faced with the demands of the canning and preserving industry (and that means you and me in the long run), are under constant pressure to produce more succulent, fibre-reduced vegetables. Tomatoes and carrots are certainly less fibrous than they used to be, since the introduction of new seed types, and no doubt this goes for some other cultivated vegetables too.

So to sum up, plant fibre is a part of our food that has long been ignored. For years it has been thought to be a waste product and treated accordingly. We now know that there's a whole family of plant fibres, each having its own unique properties, probably including many we don't yet know about. The things we do know, though, seen to indicate that fibre is a far more complicated and valuable food than we ever dreamt of. It therefore clearly deserves to be far more thoroughly researched.

This doesn't mean, of course, that refined or fibre-free foods are intrinsically bad. We simply have to be practical and see how far we can refine them before making problems for ourselves. As society is organised today it would be impossible to do without some food processing and refining, as we shall now see.

5 What have they done with our fibre?

The manipulation and processing of food is nothing new, yet it's still an emotive subject and likely to provoke anguished cries along the lines: 'What are they doing to our food, it's not what it used to be!'

Of course it's not – but nor is society. As we've already seen, man started on the road to food processing the day he left the land to live in towns. Even before then, people were undoubtedly looking for ways of preserving food, for it is by its very nature an unstable commodity. As long as 4000 years ago people were sun-drying fish and meat, and dried fruit was popular in very ancient times. Dried soups have been around for 200 years and were taken by Captain Cook on his voyage in 1772.

As the population of the West increased by leaps and bounds, ways had to be found of feeding enormous populations on food which had travelled not just the length of the country but possibly half way round the world. Cans were first used in 1812, when the Army and Navy led the way in what was probably the greatest single revolution in food technology ever. But although canned foods were available to the forces, they were very rarely found in civilian shops at that time. Then with the end of the 19th century came the introduction of refrigeration. The first successful sea voyage with a cargo of refrigerated meat was as recent as 1880.

Closely linked to improved methods of transport and storage was the use of preservatives. Salt, nitre and vinegar had been used over the centuries to preserve foods, but it wasn't until the 1880s that food preservatives as we know them were introduced. Part of the emotional outcry today against 'them' for tampering with our foods is doubtless of historical origin.

Food adulteration has been with us for centuries. Manufacturers and distributors have always tried to make their food more palatable, better looking or longer lasting by one means or another. In 1880 Accum, a food analyst, brought to light all manner of food horrors and exposed them to the public gaze. He showed how alum was being used to improve inferior grades of flour; took the lid off the wine faking trade; proved that beer makers were tainting their products with chemicals and that there was too much lead in cider and wine; and claimed that sweets had poisonous salts in them.

Things got so bad as a result of a *Lancet* article in 1850, that a select Parliamentary Committee on food adulteration was set up and the first Food and Drugs Act was passed in 1860. Under this Act official analysts were appointed, but many didn't take up their posts and of those that did, most did nothing at all. They were simply a sop to public opinion and in 1862 only 300 analytical examinations were carried out on food in the whole of England.

Ironically, it took the introduction of manufactured foods to raise standards and eliminate the dangerous practices that had gone on for centuries. Without manufactured food, with its accompanying uniformity of quality and texture, its availability throughout the year and its hygienic preparation, life as we know it today would scarcely be possible.

Manufactured, 'instant' foods are now virtually an essential part of modern life. For it's all very well pretending that we in the West could live on 'good wholesome foods' like our grandparents did – it's unlikely that we would. Modern foods mirror modern thinking and lifestyles. Only large commercial organisations are capable of growing, buying, storing, processing and marketing foods for the avid millions in the West, and businesses have to make profits. To do this they must produce what people want, whether it's best for them or not. In an ideal world this shouldn't be the case, but unless we are prepared to go back to producing our own food, we shall have to be governed to some extent by what the masses want – or pay extra for being different.

Today's housewife wants freedom from vegetable growing,

preparing and even cooking. Gone are the days when a woman was happy to spend much of her day preparing food, and domestic help is a thing of the past. And this has inevitably encouraged the food processing industry to make great strides towards simpler and easier foods at every stage.

The trouble is that in order to give foods an almost indefinite shelf or freezer life, you have to do things to them. You have to take some things away and add others. Of all the things that are taken away, dietary fibre is by far the most important. This removal of fibre we call refining, and the fibre-depleted foods so produced are called refined foods.

The two most highly refined foods we eat in the West are sugar and white flour. Because there is much more fibre in sugar beet or cane than there is proportionately in wheat grain, sugar, as it appears on our tables, is even more highly purified or refined than white flour. White sugar has almost no fibre in it at all, and indeed other sugars are just as bad. Some people assume that brown sugar is better for them because it looks more 'natural'. This is unfortunately not so: all sugar products are very highly refined and to all intents and purposes contain no fibre.

The milling of wheat (described at greater length in chapter six) involves the grinding of grain between rollers and subsequent sieving off of the germ and husk (bran). Even light milling removes most of the bran and it is this bran which contains the essential dietary fibre. Flour containing as much as 90 per cent of the original grain has already lost most of its bran because the bran, being the outermost coat of the wheat, gets milled off at the very first stage. Man has been trying to refine wheat for centuries so that it'll keep better and be easier to eat, and white flour has always been associated with purity and has been highly sought after by the rich through the ages. It has become both more popular and more widely available since 1880 and the introduction of the roller mill, and the amount of fibre consumed in bread has fallen to less than a third of what it was a century ago. This fall is accounted for partly by a drop in bread consumption, and partly by the lower proportion of fibre as bran in white bread when compared with that in 1860–70. Bread was the major source of calories in England in the early part of the last century, when the average Briton was eating 360 lb a year. By 1880 this had fallen to 280 lb and by 1970 to 145 lb.

As flour consumption fell, so did that of potatoes (from 296 lb per person per year in 1880 to 224 lb in 1970) which are also a rich source of fibre. But parallel with these falls was a rise in the consumption of fruit and vegetables. These were rare commodities until the 18th century, unless one was fortunate enough to have a garden or knew someone who had one.

The 19th century saw a small increase in fruit and vegetable consumption, but between 1909 and 1970 fruit and vegetable intake doubled in the UK, USA, Norway and Holland. Today we get most of our fibre from fruit, vegetables and nuts whereas bread and flour products account for only 13 per cent of it.

Overall then, our intake of fibre may not have changed much in the last 100 years, but what has happened is that our cereal fibre consumption has fallen considerably compared with 100 years ago. It's this fall in cereal fibre, which is especially active physiologically in the body, that we're particularly concerned about.

Most convenience foods today are refined. Even 'fresh' fruit and vegetables are so peeled and mutilated by the housewife as to make a nonsense of the fruit and vegetable fibre figures quoted in the learned journals. More and more vegetables and fruits are being grown and selected for their ease of freezing and canning, and few of us eat fruit and vegetables in their truly natural state. Even boiling for ˙ong periods (as the English seem so keen on doing) probably alters the dietary fibre content of these foods. So what with the intrinsically lower fibre content of vegetables specially bred with the food processing industry in mind, and the modern housewife's treatment of them when she does use them, it's unlikely that a doubling of the amount of fruit and vegetables consumed over the last 70 years has in fact doubled the amount of fibre we're eating from this source.

Cereal products like bread, pastries, biscuits and breakfast cereals are almost all made from highly refined white flour. White bread is a wonderful product of modern food technology and has been tailor-made for the modern housewife. Unfortunately it contains very little dietary fibre. When white flour is produced the nutritious germ and bran are sieved off, so that most of the vitamins, minerals and other valuable constituents are lost. Some of these the modern miller adds back, but as has been shown in animal experiments, simply putting things back is *not* the same as never having removed them in the first place. White bread stores well, but has all sorts of chemicals in it to ensure that it does so. It's as white and spongey as it is for the same reason. But the public has become used to white bread and feels that wholemeal bread is only for 'health-foodnuts'. There are signs that attitudes are changing however, and there is a growing interest in brown breads, which is partly due at least to an interest in healthier foods, if only in the simple belief that brown bread is better than white. This is not necessarily so. Many brown breads are simply white bread that has been coloured, and many health-orientated breads are simply such breads that have had some of the wheatgerm (removed by milling and sieving) added back. Bread like this does not compare with wholemeal bread and mustn't be confused with it.

The simplest way of ensuring a high-fibre intake is to eat wholemeal bread only, and to use wholemeal flour for all cooking. In this way you can be sure that you're getting all the fibre and all the nutrients in the grain. Some time ago an experiment was carried out in the south-east of England in which a large and expensive advertising campaign was mounted to persuade people to buy wholemeal bread. According to the white flour millers, this was unsuccessful and confirmed their conviction that people didn't want wholemeal bread. The manufacturers of wholemeal flour tell a very different story – they simply can't make enough to keep up with public demand. One company is even exporting wholemeal pasta to Italy, it's proving so popular there. The truth behind the so-called unpopularity of wholemeal bread is that it doesn't keep as well as white bread and so has to be delivered more frequently by the baker. Clearly, the bread industry doesn't want to encourage this trend. Wholemeal bread is also very much more filling to eat, because the fibre absorbs so much more water and swells in the stomach, so that you need less of it to feel full.

So the bakers would find themselves delivering less bread but more frequently to the supermarkets if wholemeal bread caught on in a big way. This is a change they are unlikely to welcome!

But some people eat no bread at all today – they eat crisp-breads and breakfast cereals instead. If the crispbreads are made with whole grain, and many are, then they are just as good as wholemeal bread as a source of fibre. But the breakfast cereals are another story. / weearaloix Ru-Bran.

Many breakfast cereals are highly refined and have little food value, while others add insult to injury by coating the fibre-depleted flakes with refined sugar.

Recently, the breakfast food industry has realised that the public are interested in a healthy diet and as a result have come up with bran-enriched cereals and muesli-type foods, which are now a multi-million-pound business. The bran-containing breakfast foods are excellent, and there is little to beat Kelloggs All-Bran (which has been available for decades) for sheer concentration of bran per spoonful – but more of this in the diet chapter later. Mueslis are good and high in fibre but should contain as little sugar as possible. Sugar, as we shall see, is an important food to restrict because it is so dangerous for teeth and such an easy way of consuming too many calories. Sugar isn't simply bad because it's had all its fibre removed. It is thought to be also actively harmful, and may play a part in producing heart disease as well as diabetes and obesity.

So we end with a dilemma. Convenience foods are here to stay, as most of us like them and find them indispensable to some degree. Yet all the signs are that – even ignoring the possible harmful effects of food colourings, additives, pre-servers, smoothing agents and so on – natural whole, un-processed foods are better for us because they contain dietary fibre. The food processing industry, contrary to popular belief, is not an ogre. We like the advantages it brings but choose to highlight the disadvantages. The answer must be to try and get the best of both worlds. After all, we can easily restore the fibre to our diets, as we shall see later.

It's unfair to say, as many do, that all processed, manufactured food is harmful. Even something as simple as table salt has additives which make it pour more easily and raise its iodine content, and few of us would be prepared to go without salt, or to put up with caked salt cellars or thyroid disease. What I will say is that it's probably wise to keep your consumption of highly manufactured foods down to a minimum, *to eat less sugar and sugar-containing foods*, and to eat high-fibre foods whenever possible.

Fortunately, the food industry itself may well provide the answer to the problem it has created on our behalf. Food manufacturers are already making high-fibre biscuits and tablets. As the public's awareness of fibre is heightened there will be an ever-increasing demand for high-fibre products and new types of high-fibre foods are undoubtedly just around the corner. Coupled with this pressure, food industry giants are beginning to realise that the millions of tons of fibre they throw away every year could and should be put to good use. So after centuries of refining our foods we may now be on the way back to a more natural, healthier diet in the West.

6 The discovery of fibre

The term 'dietary fibre' was only formally adopted in the early 1970s, so the average reader could be forgiven for thinking that this is a book about a new substance.

This is far from the case. The concept of roughage in our food and the dangers of its removal date back to Hippocrates, who found that white flour bound up the bowels in patients with diarrhoea. At this time, upper-class Greeks and Romans wanted purer flour, and indeed the Romans are said to have introduced millstones for grinding flour. This stoneground flour was then sieved to make it whiter and supposedly purer.

For centuries the fibre story has centred on bread. This is because bread was, until the 19th century, the staple food in Britain, so people were naturally interested in it. Most of the poor ate little but bread in the Middle Ages, when bread was baked in the manorial oven. The story of fibre begins with the obsession of the rich with whiter bread which, they reasoned, would be free from impurities.

Linked to their concern for the colour of bread was their worry about its adulteration by the millers and bakers of the day, who would go to almost any lengths to produce whiter bread. There were, for years, two bakers' companies – the White and the Brown Bakers. They were incorporated in 1307, but took 200 years to unite.

Quality control in milling and baking has always been a moot point. As long ago as the reign of King John we find records on the punishments meted out to unsatisfactory bakers. A careless or a dishonest baker might be 'drawn upon a hurdle from Guildhall to his own house, through the streets with his loaf hanging round his neck'. The Assize of Bread of 1266 held good until 1822, when the first Bread Act replaced it.

Bread at this time was white, brown or black, but even the best quality white flour was still very dark by today's standards because methods of milling were still simple, and the sieving of the ground-up grains so incomplete. Brown bread was in fact what we would call wholemeal bread today, and the white bread was a dirty brown.

The other great sources of dietary fibre – fruit and vegetables – were very hard to come by before the 19th century. Fruit and vegetables were only available if you had a garden or access to one, because the transport of vegetables and fruit over long distances was almost impossible. In fact, in the 11th, 12th and 13th centuries fruits were believed to produce illnesses and so were avoided. This belief is hardly surprising, because fruits were of course available in the summer, the very time when infections were rife in the community. Moreover, the people of the day confused the laxative effect of fruit and vegetables with dysentry.

Medieval physicians thought dark breads were 'poorly digested' and so did not recommend them. Thomas Cogan (1584) wrote 'Browne bread ... having much branne ... fylleth the belly with excrements and shortly descendeth the stomach.'

The tide was turning against dark breads, and because the ordinary working man wanted to emulate the rich he started to give them up in the 18th century. Soon, dark breads became equated with times of shortage.

By the 18th century bread was becoming an expensive commodity. A loaf in 1796 cost 1s 1½d so people wanted 'good' bread for their money. In 1771, Arthur Young commented that 'rye and barleybread at present are looked upon with a sort of horror by poor cottagers'. But the quality of bread generally was falling and this led the government of the day to introduce 'standard' bread from which less bran was removed. This, of course, made it darker and although it was a penny cheaper, it was very unpopular.

Because the millers couldn't produce really white flour at this time, bakers resorted to all kinds of measures to make bread white and so more acceptable. In the 1750s, bread was being whitened with chalk, alum and even ground-up bones from graveyards. This soon got the millers and bakers a bad name as rascals and villains, and controversy raged over the adulteration of bread for 50 years.

Around this time the attitude towards vegetables was slowly changing. W. Smith in his *A sure guide in sickness and Health* (1776) wrote 'a large quantity of vegetables should be constantly mixed with animal food to take off its putrescency and to prevent it from corrupting while it continues in the stomach. In short, we should eat in great moderation and make vegetables the principal part of our food.' This could be more easily done at this time as fruit and vegetables were more readily available – but still nothing like as freely available as they are today.

In the 19th century most Europeans, apart from the English, still ate rye and other dark breads. A French physiologist of the time, Magendie, did some remarkable experiments to show that dogs lived for a long time in good health when fed on coarse, dark bread and water, but became ill and died in less than two months if the bread was made from white, high-grade flour. This was possibly the first laboratory experiment looking into the action of fibre, although it must be stressed that it wasn't until the last thirty years that we've realised that the lack of *fibre* was so very important. From ancient times until the early decades of this century people were only really concerned with the nutritive parts of foods. And the constant quest for knowledge about the nourishing parts of foods meant that the fibre content was never even considered.

In 1860 a French food chemist – the inventor of margarine – made a machine for removing the outer coat of wheat, so making the grain free from bran altogether. He claimed that his end product had all the nutritive value of wheat. But his invention came to nothing, just one of many such inventions to make stone-ground flour purer. Until then stone-ground flour had been sieved or 'bolted' through finer and finer fabrics (even silk gauze sometimes) so as to remove any signs of coarseness.

The revolution came with the invention of the roller mill in 1870. Until this time grain had been milled between stones, the flour collected and then sieved through fine or coarse cloths to give the colour of flour desired. Stones were thought to be inefficient grinding surfaces, so iron rollers were introduced and patented as early as 1753. Methods changed little until 1870 when porcelain rollers were introduced. The millers loved them. They meant fast, easy milling with little upkeep (stones had to be 'dressed', a tedious hand preparatory job, before milling), and with vastly improved control of the type of flour.

There was yet another bonus. In stone grinding, the germ of the wheat, containing the valuable proteins, fats, salts and minerals, was ground up with the whole grain. With roller milling the germ was flattened into a small cake which was sifted out with the bran. This meant that the flour kept better in storage because it had no fat to go rancid. So at last the millers had a way of making very white, storable flour in large quantities – and cheaply. But even then the bread wasn't thought to be white enough, and it was treated with oxidising agents, chlorine and other bleaches before being put on sale.

At this time the main customers were the urban poor, the products of the industrial revolution and the great move of populations from country to town from the first half of the 19th century. A study of poor children in Bethnal Green, London, in 1892 found that they were nourished almost entirely on bread. 83 per cent of them had no other solid food for 17 out of 21 meals each week. The whole population was still eating a great deal of bread (about 1 lb per head per day), although middle-class workers were starting to eat meat more than bread for the first time in the country's history. But the poor of the late 19th and early 20th centuries were still living on bread and tea.

In 1837 Sylvester Graham, working in America, published a book which established him as 'the greatest apostle of Whole-meal Bread as a natural food'. The book stirred up a lot of interest and although his ideas were sponsored by a society called the Bread Reform League, he was highly regarded as an independent thinker. He it was who influenced one of the great pioneers in England – Dr T. R. Allinson. Qualifying in Medicine at the age of 23, Allinson, a vegetarian like Graham, started experimenting with the effects of diet on disease. His first article appeared in the *British Medical Journal* of December 1883. Instead of medicines he gave his patients bottles of coloured water (a placebo), but also gave them careful instructions on how to change their diet. He soon found that his patients recovered more quickly on his dietetic treatment than if he had given them medicine. On this experience much of his subsequent theory of nutrition was to be built.

Allinson was a prolific writer and an original thinker. It's worth quoting some of his book *The Advantages of Wholemeal Bread* here because it shows that he was on the track of dietary fibre without knowing it, a long time before anybody else.

We will now consider the advantage of wholemeal bread over the white loaf. The first solid food a child should have is wholemeal bread and milk, as such will aid the teeth in coming through and if a child is given no other bread but this, he can grow up tall, strong, well and cheerful. By acting as a corrector and regulator of the bowels it prevents children from being troubled with falling of the bowel or similar complaints. Growing children should all have it, as it helps to prevent their teeth from decaying early, supplies their systems with bony matter, so that they grow up of proper height . . . Grown up persons must eat this bread always, as it gives more satisfaction; hunger is not felt so readily, as it 'stays' the body better. Constipation is almost unknown amongst regular eaters of it; this complaint is accompanied by indigestion, want of energy, back-ache, weariness, dullness, depression and a dozen little ailments that do not make us ill, but yet life is not as pleasant as it might be if these were not present. Wholemeal bread, by curing this condition, does away with these distressing symptoms. Piles or haemorrhoids, varicose veins, varicocele and other like ailments are banished by it as these are caused in great measure by costive bowels . . .

Old people should always eat this bread, as it prevents constipation; this is always bad but is worse in the old, as the straining at stool may cause rupture of a blood vessel in the brain; then they have what is known as a stroke, or apoplectic fit, and if not killed outright, they are more or less crippled for life . . .

It is thus seen that Wholemeal Bread is a necessity for all classes of the community. The rich should eat it, so that it may carry off some of their superfluous foods and drinks; and the poor must eat it, then they will not need to buy so much flesh foods and other expensive articles of diet. If a law could be passed forbidding the separation of the bran from the fine flour, it would add very greatly to the health and wealth of our nation and lessen considerably the receipts of the publican, tobacconist, chemist, doctor and undertaker

. . . to banish the white flour loaf from his home is the duty of every good citizen.

Dr Allinson felt so strongly about food that he spent a great deal of his time writing about it for the public. This, and his condemnation of drugs, made an enemy of the British Medical Association and led to his being struck off the Register. After an expensive legal battle he decided to call it a day and bought up a mill in London's east end. Now he could control the content of his own bread, and for those who couldn't get to his bakery he was able to provide good wholemeal flour in a prepackaged form so that they could make their own bread.

But for all this, very few other doctors agreed with him and it really wasn't until the 1920s, when distinguished doctors such as Sir Robert McCarrison and Professor Aithur Rendell-Short wrote about the role of food in diseases, that roughage began to be of real medical interest. Rendell-Short pointed out that appendicitis was caused by a lack of roughage in the early 1920s, but very few people heeded his warning.

Before we get too deeply involved in the story since then, it might be valuable to say a few words about food research. Doctors like Allinson were, and still are, very rare birds indeed. Since the Middle Ages, doctors have had a strange professional relationship with food in general. Until comparatively recently food biochemistry was of course a closed book, and just how food actually did anything in or to the body was unknown. In the 19th and 20th centuries scientists and nutritionists especially have furthered our understanding of food, but apart from a few distinguished exceptions doctors are and always have been singularly disinterested in the food we eat.

Certainly, medical schools the world over teach the rudiments of food values, nutrition and quite a lot of detailed biochemistry. But overall, it's probably fair to say that the average medical student learns precious little about food. Indeed, nutrition is a highly unfashionable subject in medical circles – or it was until recently

The nutritional problems this century in the West have been thought to be caused by too much food while those of the rest of the world are thought to be due to its shortage. Individual diet-linked diseases have, of course, interested doctors for years and scurvy, kwashiorkor, beri-beri and many others are now treatable and preventable conditions. But these are obviously *medical* conditions presenting as *diseases* which doctors are in business to diagnose and treat. Another way of looking at the problem though is to take a leaf out of the vets' book and look at food much more carefully on the input side rather than simply to treat disease processes as they occur. We're probably a lot more careful about what we feed our animals than we are over what we eat ourselves.

Man's diet has developed somewhat haphazardly in the West since the latter part of the 19th century, as we saw in chapter three. Only now is the medical profession beginning to ask if this is safe – let alone desirable. So it's against this background that we have to view the discovery of dietary fibre this century.

The 1930s saw the first in-depth, academic interest in roughage when the Kellogg Company of Michigan sponsored several studies in the USA. Isolated workers had been looking at certain aspects of roughage but not until the Michigan State College studies were they put on to a proper scientific footing. Kelloggs were interested, quite naturally, in the effects of their product All-Bran on the bowel. The studies showed that it did have a profound laxative effect and that bran or another source of fibre was essential in preventing constipation. They studied the speeds at which food passed through the intestine and found that bran speeded up the passage of the food considerably. Undoubtedly, a lot of useful discoveries were made by these researchers, but the medical profession, both in the USA and Great Britain, didn't take them any further.

This lack of interest can be put down to several factors. First, doctors in general find such subjects rather dull and the weighing and examining of stools isn't exactly the most glamorous part of medical research! Second, some people felt that the host of scientific papers produced by the Michigan team contained claims which were too good to be true. Third, the research, though formalising what had been known for years, didn't produce anything of shattering medical importance; and fourth, a prominent American physician was arguing very persuasively at the time that man was not a herbivore and couldn't and shouldn't, be eating fibre at all.

So roughage in the diet became a non-U subject and thousands of doctors advised patients with bowel troubles to eat *low*-roughage diets.

Remember that food values were still the main concern of doctors involved with food, and with the coming of World War Two this concern took on an even deeper significance. There were severe food shortages in Britain during wartime, so the nutritionists of the day were charged with making the most of the foods available. Part of their effort included the introduction of National Flour in 1941. This was flour with a high level of fibre, or in other words flour which was not as refined as normal. In this way there was less wastage of the wheat available, because more of the grain was used and the final bulk thereby increased.

At that time scientists weren't concerned with the bran content but only with the nutritional value of this staple wartime food. In fact, although it wasn't remarked upon at the time, analysis of the fibre content of National Flour showed that there was a five-fold rise when compared with the white flour of the day. As this fibre level went up, we were also eating less of other types of food and these two factors together produced a fall in the incidence of many of the diseases so prevalent at that time. Discussions of these disease changes can be found in their respective chapters.

The Second World War threw up a vital new personality in the fibre story, every bit as important as Allinson in his day. This was Surgeon Captain T. L. Cleave.

As senior medical officer on board the battleship King George V, Captain Cleave found that the majority of the men were constipated and were suffering accordingly. Because other remedies were either unavailable or too expensive, he fed them miller's bran. As this couldn't be classed as a drug the seamen had to pay for it – which they did happily. In fact, on one occasion when the supply of bran failed, the men fell in before the captain and demanded their bran. A bold move in wartime!

To many other doctors this would have been success enough, but not to Captain Cleave. He built up a philosophy of medicine over the next 14 years as a result of his experience in many parts of the world, until in 1956 he published what is now considered to be *the* original paper on refined carbohydrates and disease. Unfortunately, it was published in a journal not seen by many doctors and its importance was missed for several more years. In this article Cleave put forward his theory that man had, for centuries, tried to be clever at Nature's expense and now he was paying for it. He laid the blame for many of our modern illnesses fairly and squarely at the feet of the food processing industry. His argument was that man had evolved over thousands of years so as to be able to eat unrefined foods, and that by usurping Nature by extracting and purifying foods he would eventually bring about his own downfall.

The main foods Cleave was concerned about were the refined carbohydrates, especially sugar and white flour. He particularly spelled out the dangers of refined sugar consumption but in this he was not alone. Doctors and nutritionists had been worried about sugar since the turn of the century and Dr Paten, a physician at St Andrew's, Scotland, wrote learned and well-documented articles on the evils of sugar in the Edinburgh Medical Journal of 1932. He pointed to the unnaturalness of eating a purified, manufactured chemical such as sugar; to the changes it caused in digestion; to the possibility that it could produce vitamin deficiencies, diabetes, catarrh and increased tumour growth rates.

So it's probably fair to say that Surgeon Captain Cleave didn't actually produce anything new as such, but rather that he pulled together many loose ends and by doing so made people sit up and take notice. He showed that refining foods meant consuming less fibre, and he produced many convincing arguments to back his hypothesis. This may sound as though it was easy. It wasn't. It meant 25 years of careful clinical research, culminating in the publication in 1966 of his book *Diabetes, Coronary Thrombosis and the Saccharine Disease*. In the foreword to the second edition Sir Richard Doll wrote that if only a small part of the predictions made in the book proved to be correct, '. . . the author will have made a bigger contribution to medicine than most university departments or medical research units make in the course of a generation'.

This book triggered off new ideas in the minds of other physicians and surgeons the world over, and so must be considered a medical landmark.

But to be fair, medical history is rarely made by one man alone. In the late 1940s, Dr A. R. P. Walker, working in South Africa, was looking into fibre and its effects in considerable detail. His early studies showed that prisoners eating wholemeal bread suffered from considerably less appendicitis and heart disease than their fellows in the outside world. Since then he and his research unit have worked untiringly to prove and reprove the effects of a high-fibre diet on the bowel in many different races. Dr Walker is probably the greatest single repository of knowledge on the subject of fibre living today. He has devoted more than 30 years to painstaking research, research without which this book, for instance, would be impossible.

But books by Captain Cleave and work by Dr Walker in Africa, however valuable, could make little impact on the world until the medical profession and the public could be fired with enthusiasm for the fibre story.

The first foundation stone for this enthusiasm was laid in 1964 by Mr Neil Painter – a London surgeon. Painter had written a thesis two years previously in which he reported that the pressures inside the bowels of patients with diverticular disease (the commonest disease of the colon after constipation) were abnormally high. In 1964 he took the bold step of defying the medical teaching of decades by writing that low-roughage foods were *bad* for the bowel. In the years that followed he put patients on bran because he argued that constipation, which Cleave had shown was prevented by bran, was closely related to diverticular disease.

After several years' experience with diverticular disease patients on bran, he was ready in 1971 to publish his conclusion that bran and high-roughage diets were not only *harmless* –

they were actually beneficial. So for the first time a respected practising surgeon, no armchair theoretician, had turned this basic medical principle on its head. This may not seem very dramatic to a layman, but when you learn that in the years immediately leading up to this several top physicians were in practice using high-fibre diets but dared not let it be known for fear of ridicule – you'll see how bold a step it was.

The second essential foundation stone came in the shape of Mr Denis Burkitt, who had already carved a niche for himself in the medical history books by describing a common but hitherto unrecognised cancer in African children, later named after him. Burkitt was not only a household name in medicine: he brought to the subject of dietary fibre a zeal and enthusiasm that has infected doctors the world over. He was just what the fibre story needed – a distinguished clinician, with a quarter of a century's experience in those countries in which our Western diseases are rare, and a magnificent public relations man. Since Burkitt's entry into the fibre field less than ten years ago he has not only acted as a catalyst and coordinator but has also collected vast amounts of data from his worldwide contacts which have helped to further our understanding of the subject.

But like any discovery there are other no less important figures working on various specific facets of the fibre story, although they may not hit the headlines as often as the ones I've mentioned already. Dr Kenneth Heaton of Bristol Royal Infirmary has ten years of gallstone and fibre research behind him; Dr Martin Eastwood of Edinburgh, 15 years of looking at fibre and bile acids; Dr Hugh Trowell, 30 years of epidemiological research into the pattern of diseases in Africans – and there are many more. The fibre story may only just have become a reality to the public and indeed to most of the medical profession; but pioneers like these have been building on Surgeon Captain Cleave's original work for many years. So it's no five minute wonder or 'food fad' that will go away if you wait long enough. Today, scarcely a week goes by without some new research being announced, and work is now under way in scores of centres the world over.

As Sir Richard Doll, Regius Professor of Medicine at the

University of Oxford, wrote in a foreword to Burkitt and Trowell's medical textbook *Refined Carbohydrate Foods and Disease*, 'Once every ten years or so a new idea emerges about the cause of disease that captures the imagination and, for a time, seems to provide a key to the understanding of many of those diseases whose cause was previously unknown ... To these we may now add a deficiency of dietary fibre.'

Section two
Fibre and disease

7 Dental caries . . . the tooth, the tooth and nothing but

If you want to see the commonest disease in the Western world today, go to a mirror and open your mouth. If you're one of the three in a thousand who *hasn't* got dental decay – you're lucky. The statistics show that if you're over fifty you'll have lost half your teeth already, indeed half of all fifty-year-olds have no teeth at all.

Dental decay and the gum disease that so often accompanies it are a scourge of epidemic proportions in the West. By the age of five, children have on average five decayed, missing or filled (DMF) teeth and dental disease costs the nation more to treat than any other, with the exception of mental ill-health. On top of this nearly half the population over sixteen has some false teeth – a frightening thought.

The trouble is that we have come to accept, quite wrongly, that dental decay and tooth loss are inevitable. They're not. Tooth decay and gum disease are relatively 'new' diseases brought upon ourselves by eating the wrong food.

Dental caries was almost unknown in Ancient Man for nearly a million years, and is still rare today in a few areas of the world. Obviously it's difficult to know exactly what the caries rate was hundreds or even thousands of years ago but careful studies have been done which bring to light some remarkable facts.

First of all let's be clear how we know whether teeth were lost from an ancient skull before or after the owner's death. If a tooth is lost before death the bony socket grows over again whereas if the tooth falls out after death the socket remains 'open'. Armed with this information, researchers examined skulls from ancient graves. Professor J. L. Hardwick compared 1014 teeth in Anglo-Saxon skulls with the same number of matched teeth in 1957. He found caries in 9·5 per cent of the old skulls and in 48·6 per cent of the modern ones.

A study of 199 sets of jawbones from the skeletons in the cemetery of St Leonard's Church, Hythe, all originating from 1250–1650, showed that about half the owners had not lost a single tooth. Similar studies of a burial ground in Farringdon Street, London, found that 26 per cent of males and 14·5 per cent of females had all their teeth when they died. Not only did all these skulls have more teeth than would be found today but of those remaining, only ten per cent were carious. Just compare this with the situation today in the West, when only seven in 100 people between the ages of 25 and 35 have all their teeth, and you'll soon agree that there's been a dramatic increase in dental disease over the centuries.

Today the average adult in the West has about 16 DMF (decayed, missing or filled) teeth compared with two in most primitive rural populations of the world, and about the same again in ancient man. Rural populations have been studied in Alaska, India, Kenya, Mexico, Peru, Uganda and many other countries and their low level of caries documented.

But before we go on to see exactly why we have so much dental disease, let's see what causes it.

Dental caries is by and large a disease of Western civilisations and starts with a microscopic layer of protein which is deposited on the teeth from saliva. This is called *pellicle* and soon becomes impregnated with organisms (also from saliva) to form a new substance called *plaque*. Plaque is a thick, sticky slime which forms on our teeth all the time and depends for its existence on the sugar in our food. The sugar we eat helps feed the bacteria in the plaque and it's these bacteria which produce acids which make holes in teeth.

Dental caries was thought for years to be a fairly straightforward process, but recent research has proved otherwise. It now seems that because of our high sugar intake (the average Westerner eats in two weeks what an Elizabethan took a year to eat) plaque is forming all the time on our teeth. As it gets thicker it sticks more firmly to the teeth and if it's not cleaned off every day it rots the teeth and causes gum disease too. It's recently become apparent that almost all teeth are constantly being attacked by acid bacterial products, yet for some reason not everybody gets cavities. Dental decay is a continuous, dynamic process – small cavities being created and repaired spontaneously under the right conditions. This new discovery is especially interesting because it might help us to understand why our ancestors and whole populations in the world today don't lose their teeth through decay.

So what is responsible for this epidemic of decay and gum disease in the West? There's no point beating about the bush – the answer is simple . . . *sugar*, and especially refined sugar. Sugar as we know it, is in no sense a natural food. It's a manufactured product much like plastic or paint, both of which have also come from living things just like sugar.

Because as a species we seem to like the sweet taste of sugar, it's always been in great demand. Originally, cane sugar came from India or Arabia to the West and was used for making marzipan and sweets. It had always been a luxury, up to the last 150 years or so. In fact in the 13th century loaf sugar cost five to ten pence a pound: so obviously only the rich could afford it and we find that it was they who had the decay and gum disease.

As sugar became cheaper over the years, more and more of it was eaten, until today the average Englishman eats about 120 lbs every years. The numbers of teeth lost throughout history have usually paralleled the consumption of sugar. Pretty conclusive evidence. Of course many will say that there have been a great number of enormous changes over the last 500 years other than the increased consumption of sugar, and that perhaps one of these could have made our teeth fall out. This is, of course, a perfectly reasonable suggestion but it has been ruled out by several studies done in this century.

Perhaps one of the best of these was the study of the population of Tristan da Cunha. In 1932 this previously isolated community was looked at by the surgeon of a visiting ship. He examined the teeth of 162 inhabitants in some detail, and found that 83 per cent of them were entirely free from caries and that no child under five had a single bad tooth. In addition to this the level of periodontal or gum disease was also very low.

The ship left white refined flour and sugar behind because the inhabitants liked them.

On a subsequent visit three years later the number of good teeth had fallen by more than 50 per cent. The only change in the people's diet had been in the consumption of white flour and sugar from passing ships.

Similar studies on Eskimos have shown very much the same results. In other words, there's no reason to believe that certain populations or species are immune to caries – in fact the only animal we know that is, is the monkey. If you feed refined foods and especially sugar to human beings, they get tooth decay. According to a study of a population of Eskimos, it took just ten years of sugar-eating to render the teeth of the whole population carious. And these Eskimos, just like the people of Tristan da Cunha, had no substantial change in eating habits over that period except for the consumption of white flour and sugar. So one or both of these refined foods must be to blame. But which? Some experts have maintained that white flour rather than sugar is actually the culprit.

Certainly white flour was known in Roman times, and, like 'pure' white sugar more recently, was always in demand by the richer classes that could afford it. And it has been argued that the slight increase in the numbers of teeth lost over the years before the mass consumption of sugar was due to the increased popularity of white bread. But this is now thought to be un-likely. White refined flour definitely makes bread which is sticky and more likely to remain in the crevices of the teeth and causes decay; but this alone isn't enough to cause caries. Plaque is at its most harmful when it is thick, and when it sticks firmly to the enamel surface of the tooth. The plaque which is formed by starchy foods like bread is much less sticky than that formed by sugar, and it comes away from the tooth surface much more easily. There are many areas in the world where starchy food consumption is high yet dental disease is low. Add to this the fact that white flour and wholemeal flour are almost equally caries-producing and the flour argument collapses.

Now for sugar itself. All sugars are known to be caries-producing, but sucrose is the worst offender of all. Even naturally-occurring fruit sugar causes plaque to form on the teeth, though it's very difficult to eat large quantities of this in a concentrated form because, apart from dates and raisins, most fruits don't actually contain large amounts in proportion to their weight.

It was thought until very recently that sugar was relatively harmless to the teeth if it was eaten bound up by its own fibre – that is unrefined. The West Indians were cited as supposedly having little decay although they are brought up chewing on sugar cane. It's certainly true that you'd have to eat an enormous volume of sugar cane to get the equivalent of the sugar in a bar of chocolate; but unfortunately the theory of the West Indians and their good teeth fell apart at the seams when Cuban caries was looked at by a Moscow-based research team recently. They found that the caries rate in the general population was high, contrary to popular belief, and that the level of decay and gum disease in the *macheteros*, the cane-cutters, was even higher still – due to their exceptional consumption of unrefined sugar because they were being given a bonus of cane if they worked well.

Certainly it is true that sugar 'diluted' by being bound up in a fibrous form is relatively less caries-producing than refined sugar, but that's mainly because it's difficult to take in large quantities of it – unless you're a *machetero*! After all, you have to chew your way through four large apples, which could take up to twenty minutes, in order to get the same sugar intake as drinking a small can of fizzy pop. This concentration-effect in the refining of foods is especially important when thinking about obesity, as we shall see.

But the closest correlation can be drawn between the intake of refined sugar and tooth decay. There has been a parallel in the graphs of sugar intake and dental disease for nearly two hundred years. Only in two periods during this time has the incidence of decay fallen, and these were both during the great World Wars of this century, when sugar consumption fell because of rationing. Interestingly enough there was a similar fall in decay during the second half of the 16th century, when, as a result of the increased taxes on sugar, consumption fell dramatically.

Today, the study of sugar and its effect on teeth has reached an advanced level. We now know that it's not so much what you eat but how you eat it that's the main problem. Sugar is at its most harmful if it remains in the mouth for a long time. The safest way to take sugar or sweets is to have a feast once a week and then to clean your teeth. If you keep your sugar eating down to once a day and clean your teeth afterwards, your chances of dental decay are higher than on the weekly system, but not dramatically so. But if you eat the same amount of sugar and sweets but this time between meals, that spells disaster. Not only does it provide an almost constant sugar bath for your teeth and gums, but it enables plaque to grow in its thickest, most dangerous form. Thick plaque absorbs more sugar, so producing more caries.

At one time it was thought that sugar as a chemical substance might itself be harmful to teeth, after it had been absorbed by the intestine. Experiments involving the feeding of animals by tubes direct into their stomachs, however, showed that sugar must come into direct contact with the teeth in order to produce caries. Tube-fed animals don't get dental decay, even if you feed them lots of sugar. This surface activity of sugar, refined or unrefined, is especially powerful in children. The Tristan da Cunha study showed only too well that children's teeth are most susceptible to decay and that as we get older our enamel gets more caries-resistant. Sugar can't get through the gums of a baby and damage the teeth before they come through as was thought at one time, but the day the teeth break through the gum surface they're in danger. The pernicious practice of dipping babies' dummies into honey (itself a highly refined, by the bees, sugar) and of filling comforters with sugary liquids, is in great part responsible for the enormous numbers of people with false teeth. 38 per cent of people over 16 in the UK have some kind of false teeth.

Mothers today have a great responsibility to their children, because now that we know the facts we ignore them at our peril.

But it's unfair to put the blame on mothers alone. We as a nation don't put nearly the emphasis on preventive dentistry that other countries do. In the USA and Sweden tooth decay is no longer taken as being inevitable, and the governments spend large amounts of money using television and other influential media to make people realise this. It's an enormous educational job to alter people's eating habits, but it's well worth while. In a society whose government subsidises sugar, the battle is bound to be an uphill one. The time, money and energy being literally wasted on dental care today is enormous, and this when only half the population ever goes to the dentist.

Before we look at the value of high-fibre foods in the battle against tooth decay, a word or two about periodontal or gum disease.

Generally speaking, the main dental problem in children is tooth decay because, as we've seen, the enamel of children's teeth is less resistant to caries than that of adults. In adults though, the caries rate falls off and diseases of the gums take over as the prime offenders. It's a little-known fact that more teeth are lost in the Western world through gum disease than through tooth decay.

The teeth are embedded in the bony sockets of the jaw and tethered by tiny fibres which hold the tooth and give it a small amount of 'play' in the socket when we chew. The gums themselves are firm, pink and stippled when healthy, but when they become inflamed these tiny fibres may be destroyed and the tooth becomes loosened.

The commonest cause of gum inflammation (*gingivitis*) is plaque. Not only does plaque form on the teeth in areas clearly visible to the dentist and available to the toothbrush, but it also builds up around the necks of the teeth and just inside the gum where the tooth goes in. This bacteria-laden plaque irritates the gums and produces inflammation. Plaque which is left undisturbed around the necks of the teeth hardens into tartar which in turn attracts more plaque.

Chronic inflammation of the gums is a common disease in most countries of the world, and more than 90 per cent of the population of the United Kingdom suffers from it. The incidence of periodontal disease in rural communities living on natural unrefined foods is usually low, though it varies from place to place very much more than that of caries. On the other hand many rural communities have poor gum health and lose most of their teeth from this. The pygmies of the Amazon basin are a good example. They lose almost no teeth through caries because of their traditionally sugar-free unrefined diet yet lose many teeth through gum disease.

Gum disease is apparently more marked among people eating mainly soft foods than among those eating mostly firm or hard chewy foods.

Toothbrushing not only removes plaque but also massages the gums. That's why it's so important to brush from gum to tooth tip. By massaging the gums, either with a brush or by chewing large volumes of fibrous foods (or both), the gums are kept healthy.

For years people have remarked that primitive rural tribes never use a toothbrush yet seem to have good teeth. We know that the main reason is that they don't eat refined sugar. But there may be other protective factors against caries in their water or food of which we are only just beginning to learn. Could it be that primitive peoples living on a largely unrefined diet rich in fibre clean their teeth by chewing for long periods on their hard, fibrous foods?

The answer, unfortunately, is not a simple one. Fibre-rich foods are certainly more abrasive to the tooth's surface than soft, pappy, refined foods. But the very areas where plaque causes most trouble are those places where food debris collects – in the fissures or cracks on the biting surfaces of the big back teeth, in between the teeth and under the gum edge. Unfortunately, you could chew all day on as hard and fibrous a diet as you liked and you wouldn't get those areas free of plaque simply by chewing. This is because food, however soft or hard, never gets any leverage on the plaque in these places. Fibre-rich food could play an important part in cleaning the surface of the teeth mechanically, but only if we extracted every other tooth and let it get to all the surfaces of the remaining teeth. Not many people would be keen on this!

Certainly an apple or a carrot makes the easily accessible flat surfaces of the teeth (where decay is rare) feel clean and free from plaque, but such foods don't clean the important areas. So much of the teaching of dentists themselves over the years is now seen to be misleading. But having said that, it's still important to understand that given the choice between chewing an apple or a carrot or eating a chocolate bar, the balance is infinitely in favour of the former because of the lower concentration of the sugar, and the smaller absolute amount of sugar you take in.

As anyone who has ever eaten a high-fibre diet will know, these foods take a lot of chewing. It's been suggested that the large amount of saliva produced by all this chewing helps wash the surface of the teeth, buffers any acids produced and so keeps them free from plaque. This may well be true in primitive people eating traditional diets, but it is unlikely to be of much help to anyone eating a highly refined diet. If you eat sugar in any form, thick plaque adheres to the tooth surface. Neither chewing rough foods nor the production of any amount of saliva will remove it – only a toothbrush will. In experiments in which sugar and apples were eaten, the caries-producing power of thick plaque was found to be greatest some time after eating the foods because the plaque had absorbed sugar. On the other hand, recent work has shown that saliva is effectively prevented from having any beneficial effects on the tooth if the plaque is thick (some people think there may be naturally occurring anti-caries substances in saliva). What we can say about people on high-fibre diets who eat no refined sugar is that they probably never form really thick plaque and so the beneficial washing action of saliva, the abrasive action of the food and the protective substances in the saliva at least have a chance to work.

So it's possible that fibrous foods help natural protective factors either in the saliva or in the food to get to where they're meant to act – on the surface of the enamel. Natural, unrefined foods are thought to have certain protective factors in them which stop teeth decaying, but just how they work and what they are is as yet a mystery.

Fibre-eating populations have flat grinding teeth worn away over the years because they use their teeth doing what they were made for – chewing. Our grinding back teeth on the other hand are deeply furrowed because we hardly use them for chewing at all. These furrows or fissures in our teeth are a haven for plaque, and if you look at your own teeth you'll probably find they're filled with dental amalgam. The rural dweller on his traditional diet doesn't have these fissures and so has one less site for dental decay. Incidentally, the gums round these flat grinding teeth also have less disease than our comparable gums.

In addition to all these dental advantages of eating unrefined foods there may well be others of which we as yet know nothing. As we saw in chapter four, 'What is fibre?', there are all sorts of naturally-occurring chemical substances associated with fibre of whose function we know nothing. It's quite possible that the reason that unrefined diets produce little or no caries is somehow linked to these substances themselves. The answer certainly isn't going to be a simple one. As recently as 1975 a village was found in Columbia where dental decay is almost unknown and yet the villagers consume large amounts of refined sugar. So far this is the only population in the world in which this combination has been documented. Analysis of their drinking water suggests that the chemical reactions taking place on the surface of their teeth are very different from those on ours, but no actual 'protective' factors have been isolated so far. It's certainly nothing as simple as fluoride in the water.

In summary then, what seems to be happening? If we go on as we are today in the West we'll all be wearing false teeth by the age of thirty within a few generations. False teeth, however good, are no substitute for natural teeth, and we're going to need teeth to eat even our refined sloppy food because man's gums weren't made for chewing. Aesthetically, natural teeth, well cared for, are most pleasing – and vast fortunes are spent in the West on restorative and cosmetic dentistry in an effort to mimic nature.

So the answer's simple. Even if you doubt the harm that refined foods can do in any other part of the body, I hope you're convinced that in the place the food starts its journey – the mouth – refined food starts to wreak havoc. And this is only the beginning.

8 Obesity . . . killing off the fat of the land

When did you last stand in front of your mirror and look at yourself – naked and sideways? If you haven't recently, do it today. Now preferably. Do you like what you see and if not, what are you doing about it?

If you're one of the 40 per cent of the population that's obese (technically 10 per cent above your ideal weight) you'll want to lose weight safely, quickly and as easily as possible without resorting to faddy diets you can't stick to and without being too much of a misery to yourself or to those around you. Then once you've taken off the pounds, you'll want to be able to keep them off – not just for a week or two but for good. Did you know that about 90 per cent of fat people put back on all their lost pounds and sometimes even more, especially after some of the more prohibitive diets? Did you realise that it's easier to get long-term cures for cancer than it is for obesity? A sobering thought, but the statistics don't lie.

You may want to get slim because you want to get into more up-to-date clothes, or simply because you feel and look better when you're slim – most people do. There's nothing like being fat to age someone, and many a slimmed fatty will tell you how much younger she looks, and feels, after getting rid of those extra pounds. We think people look older if they're fat because we automatically associate fatness with middle age.

This is quite an indictment in itself – after all, you never see a fat, middle-aged wild animal unless there is a real advantage in terms of survival. Thus an arctic seal feeds for only a few months a year and must store fat for survival. There's nothing *natural* about getting fat in middle age, as numerous studies from all over the world prove. It's only in the West that we seem to take this for granted. Animals quite naturally keep slim by balancing out food and exercise whatever age they are. The trouble is that we force-feed ourselves on refined foods as if we were Strasbourg geese whose livers go to make *paté de foie gras*. That's why we get middle-age spread.

So let's start off with wanting to look and stay young and take it from there. Something that goes with looking young is looking more attractive too. Even in these days of women's lib most women want to catch a man and keep him, and overall men in our Western culture aren't keen on fat women. If you're 15 stone you might do well in certain middle Eastern countries, but the average Englishman or American won't rave about you. In our Western civilisation we seem to think less harshly of a plump man than we do of a fat woman, but ideas are changing fast and overweight is becoming not only unfashionable but also unacceptable to lots of people. Employers too would rather have trim, well-groomed workers than those who look as though they can't control their eating.

But the main reason why most of us want to be slim is because we know that if we're fat we won't live as long as we could, and we'll get all kinds of trouble thin people aren't bothered by nearly so much. There are lots of health problems linked with obesity: to give you just an idea, bear in mind that fat people have more diabetes, gallbladder trouble, varicose veins, backache, blood pressure, heart disease and infertility than their thin brothers and sisters. If that isn't enough to convince you that it's worth sparing your body the enormous ball and chain of fat you're dragging around, I don't know what is.

'But,' I can hear you say, 'I'm not an enormous barge, I'm only a few pounds overweight.' So you may be, but remember that obesity is like pregnancy – you can't have a touch of it. If you're too heavy, you're too heavy. No ifs or buts, you've just got to do something about it. Statistics from the Metropolitan Life Assurance Company show that a man over the age of 45 decreases his survival chances by 8 per cent for every 10 lb he is overweight. So if you're 50 lb overweight, and many thousands of people are, you're increasing your chances of dying prematurely by over 40 per cent.

The thing is that the way you get rid of 5 lb is exactly the same as the way you get rid of 50 lb, and you'll soon see how. In fact 5 lb is just as important as 50 lb or even more so. You can't build a house without a foundation and those first few pounds are your foundation for being fat.

Unfortunately, these foundations are laid in childhood and are difficult to eradicate. It's widely accepted that obesity starts very early in infancy. In many post-natal wards, the very first thing a child is given is a drink of glucose water, so his introduction into the world goes hand in hand with refined carbohydrate intake! Babies quickly become used to sweet foods and soon won't take anything unless it is sweet. Sugar and other refined foods start children off on the downward spiral of more food, more weight, and earlier death as adults. Some authorities have shown that fat cells, once created in the infant, never actually disappear. They may be full or empty of fat, but they're always there. This has led one British paediatrician to coin the phrase 'Fat babies produce young widows' – quite a depressing thought. But obesity among the young is now a disease of epidemic proportions – the happy thing is that it's a preventable one.

Most people reading this chapter will be tired by now of hearing themselves making excuses and working out alibis like a hardened criminal. You can spend only so long talking about the mitigating circumstances, the glands, the family tendency to overweight, the 'inhuman demands' your body makes for food, your metabolism, your worries and so on. There are obviously a few people who do have a serious underlying medical problem which makes them fat, but of the millions of obese people this group forms less than 1 per cent. *All the rest have simply eaten the wrong foods.*

In Biblical times, fatness went with plenty and only the rich could afford highly refined foods. To be fat then was to be a living testament to your wealth and standing in society. Today, if you're fat, you pay for it – literally – because the Life Insurance companies *weight* (a very appropriate term!) their premiums if you are obese.

Over the years, fatness has been linked with happiness. This was probably because fat (that is wealthy) people actually were happier overall than the wretches who begged from them, but the image has stuck.

The myth that fat people are happy people is still very much in evidence today when people still overfeed their babies because they think they are happier if they are rounder . . . little do they know.

Just look at some of the most successful painters of the last few hundred years – they didn't paint thin women. Rembrandt, Botticelli and Rubens' women all had rounded, chubby figures and by today's standards would have been called fat. So here again overweight was linked to happiness and glamour.

As recently as Victorian times the good English matronly figure was held in esteem by almost everybody. The ideal mother was, by definition, rather round and 'stately'. This again was very much a hangover from the rich middle and upper classes, who were constantly gorging themselves. Twenty-course meals were not uncommon in a good upper class home at this time, and often guests would retire graciously to vomit so as to make room for more!

Other areas of the world, even today, still regard fatness as a very desirable thing, especially in their women. Some African pastoral tribes insist on their women being enormously fat and one chief at the end of the last century fed his wives, by force if necessary, with milk and cream so that they were so fat they could only grovel on the floors of their huts all day. A thin girl probably had tuberculosis, also common in their cattle and in their children. Thinness was feared.

The point is that this is not at all typical of Africa today or even then, or indeed of any other predominantly rural community anywhere in the world. People in such communities tend to be slim and obesity is remarkable when it occurs.

So when Dr Hugh Trowell, a key figure in the fibre story, returned to Africa after many years and saw numbers of fat Africans as he alighted from his aircraft, he could scarcely believe it was the same country that he had lived in for so many years. The answer of course was that he was looking at the urbanised Africans who had taken on our Western way of life, and with it our Western diseases.

Primitive man on a natural unrefined diet was almost certainly not overweight, and now we've come through the 'food is wealth' era, we should be able to settle down to regarding slimness as the norm in our culture – which of course it can be. Human beings if left to eat natural foods, living in as far as possible natural surroundings, do *not* get fat. Overweight is a disease we have brought upon ourselves, so we should be able to prevent it and possibly find ways to reduce its burden even in adult life.

Today we admire slimness and because we realise just how unhealthy it is to be fat, we are getting aggressive about obesity. This is a good thing. I'm not suggesting that people who are overweight should be bullied, browbeaten or cajoled – they already have enough problems and a lot more they don't even know about. No, we all have our part to play in helping people to get slim and stay slim and there's nothing like a convert to do the job.

Such converts have played an important role in the enormous growth of slimming clubs and organisations, of which there are more than 2000 in the UK alone. The British spend more than £60 million a year on slimming foods, and there has never been more interest in the subject by the press and magazine world. Yet all these 'experts' are only doing what you and I can do in our own homes – and we can do it far cheaper. Slimming has become big business and there are many who aim to keep it that way, but the money to support the slimming industry comes from only one source – you.

Slimming, done properly, is a real do-it-yourself business and doing it yourself saves time and money. Let's see how.

To understand how *roughage* helps you slim and why refined foods are so bad we need to see why we feel hungry. The simple answer is, we don't know for certain. What we do know from human and animal experiments is that there are two main sensations involved. The first is a feeling of emptiness and the second is a real sensation of hunger. Scientists have demonstrated that there is a special area of the brain called the 'appestat' which is a sort of regulator that switches our desire to eat on and off. This centre in the brain is still a medical enigma but it does help us to understand the basic concepts of appetite control.

Animals left in the wild and allowed to eat all they want don't get fat. They spend the appropriate proportion of the day eating just as much as they need, and if they get hungry they go to great lengths if necessary to satisfy their demand for food. Animals other than carnivores mostly eat natural plant foods which contain starch, sugar, fat and protein together with fibre. They never eat fibre-free foods.

If we in the West feel hungry we don't have to go to very great lengths to satisfy our appetites. We simply eat a piece of bread and butter, some instant potatoes or a chocolate bar. By doing so we take in a huge slug of calories, our blood sugar goes up and the appestat shuts down. We are happy and think all is well – but is it?

No, because within an hour we're hungry again and so have to repeat the procedure. Refined foods are almost completely absorbed so we rapidly feel empty and *are* empty. A fair portion of unrefined food remains behind and is not absorbed into the blood. This is the major shortcoming of many of the refined foods we eat – they give us a transient sense of fullness only. Because of this we eat more of them, thereby consuming enormous numbers of calories and so getting fat.

So clearly, there's something basically wrong with the type of food we eat and *not*, as is usually thought, with the amount of it. When we look at the way our intestines work it's not difficult to see where the trouble lies.

The human digestive system is a highly complicated chemical factory. From the moment food enters our mouths saliva mixes with it and starts digestion; in the stomach, acids and powerful enzymes are added; in the small intestine bile salts emulsify the fats we eat and the food is propelled along at the best possible speed, so as to ensure that the valuable food substances are absorbed into the bloodstream. The lining of the bowel absorbs nutrients in differing amounts at different places and has a lining which produces mucus to lubricate the food and protect the bowel wall. Finally, the food residue is stored in the colon, and water and chemicals are absorbed before the rest is passed as stools. The whole of this sophisticated process goes on hour after hour every day of our lives.

The reason we need so complex a system is that our food isn't in a form that the body can readily use. Every stage of digestion breaks down complex animal and plant materials into simple substances like glucose and amino acids which the body can use for energy or growth. So basically our gut does two things – it processes our food and extracts the valuable parts. But what happens if we usurp part of the bowel's function and supply it with ready-processed, partly extracted food? Will it still behave normally?

Dr Kenneth Heaton of Bristol University who did much of the original thinking on this subject uses a very helpful analogy to explain the situation.

A smelting works producing iron is normally provided with crude iron ore, that is with rocks containing various amounts of iron. The purpose of the works is to process this ore and smelt to extract the iron from it. Let us suppose that one day the lorries and trains start supplying the works with pure iron in place of some of its usual crude ore. What will happen? There would seem to be two likely consequences. (1) The output of the works will be artificially increased. As a result, stockpiles of iron will accumulate unless special efforts are made to dispose of the extra metal. (2) If the inflow of pure iron is allowed to continue, the reduction in intake of crude ore, the normal raw material, will force part of the works to shut down. This will cause unemployment and loss of morale in the workers, and may well lead to disputes and even strikes.

If we look at obesity with this in mind what we see is a huge stockpiling of energy which is turned into fat by the body. This is because the 'raw materials' our bodies were meant to consume are not being supplied. Instead, we are eating the end products of the food processing industry. Although proteins, fats and carbohydrates all produce energy when absorbed from the bowel, it is mainly carbohydrates whose properties are altered by extraction and processing and so it is with these that we are most concerned.

But cutting down calorie intake by reducing carbohydrate intake is not the only answer to obesity, because food doesn't just supply energy and building material for our bodies, it also makes us feel full.

The secret then must be to eat foods which produce a long-lasting feeling of fullness while giving enough energy and nutrients for the body to function properly. High-fibre foods do this and this is why.

Nature wraps up food materials in a protective cocoon of fibre. Just think of a sugarbeet. If we remove the fibre the final sugar is only 16 per cent of the whole weight of the original beet. So if we eat high-fibre foods we end up eating a lot of fibre in order to consume the amount of nutrients we want. This is, as far as we can tell, the way our bodies were made to take plant foods.

Because high-fibre foods need so much chewing, the amount of saliva produced in the mouth is much greater than when eating refined foods. This saliva, together with the bulky nature of high-fibre foods, produces a larger volume in the stomach which in turn makes us feel full very quickly.

So by removing the fibre from our food mechanically, we make the contained energy a great deal easier to get at and thus a lot easier for the bowel to absorb. But by removing the fibre we also remove nature's brake on overconsumption, because we remove the bulk which fills us up.

Of all the refined foods, sugar presents the greatest problem, because it can be eaten in so many concentrated forms. To take in the number of calories equivalent to those in a small bottle of pop in the form of apples, means you'd have to eat your way through four large apples. The drink would go down in two minutes but the apples would take 20 at least, and would in addition make you feel fuller.

So cutting out sugar is useful when slimming not only because by doing so you reduce your calorie intake, but also because it is just about the most highly refined of all the foods we eat. An interesting study was carried out in Capetown in which 51 office workers were asked to cut out all sugar-containing foods, but were also asked to try and keep at their present weight by eating anything else they liked. They simply couldn't do it and after five months they'd lost 3 lb on average and some as many as 5 lb. And this was while still eating a diet high in other refined foods!

Another study in Ireland involved the eating of at least 1 lb of potatoes every day. The subjects were allowed to eat whatever else they liked provided that they ate at least 1 lb of potatoes. After a few weeks they had nearly all lost weight, simply because the potatoes were so filling, since they contained such a lot of unabsorbable fibre, that the subjects had little room for anything else.

It seems that a diet devoid of all refined carbohydrates is almost bound to make you lose weight simply because you eat so many fibre-rich foods in their place.

As a bonus, it's certain that people on high-fibre, unrefined diets also absorb less of the energy they take in. Research has shown that one of the actions of fibre is that it increases the amount of energy and fat passed in the stools. Since fat is a potent source of calories this could mean that high-fibre foods help keep you slim by this action too. They may also actually prevent the complete absorption of other foods because food containing a lot of fibre passes through the bowel more quickly, so allowing less time for absorption.

Work done at Glasgow University showed that the amount of both fat and energy passed out in the stools went up as the amount of fibre in the diet was increased. Three groups of subjects were studied. The first was put on white bread with no fruit or vegetables except potatoes. The second was put on wholemeal bread with some fruit and vegetables and the third on a high-fibre diet. What they found was that the less fibre there was in the diet the more energy was extracted from the food. So it's likely that obesity is caused by getting too much out of our food. This is not only because we're eating too much but also because we're eating the wrong food.

Studies among certain rural Africans show that although they eat far greater quantities of starchy foods than we do, they still don't get fat because they're eating this starch 'wrapped up' in its natural fibre.

At this point we must just mention exercise, because people always assume that non-Westerners, especially those living in a traditional, rural way, walk enormous distances and so lose weight by exercising. This is simply not true. It's almost impossible to lose meaningful amounts of weight by exercising. True, if you take really large amounts of exercise you can lose weight, but you'd need to climb a mountain the height of Ben Nevis to work off the calories gained in a single slap-up dinner. It's also fair to say that if you're used to taking lots of exercise (as is an athlete for example), you'll probably put on weight when you give it up. This is because your body is in energy balance just as long as you keep active, but is thrown out of balance when you give up this strenuous way of life yet continue to eat the same amount of food.

Studies among prisoners and among caged animals in zoos, both of which groups have severely restricted activity, show that neither group puts on weight if its food is kept as normal.

So to sum up, our ideas on slimming have been revolutionised as our knowledge on fibre has increased. Doctors know from experience that patients cannot stick to a diet on which they feel hungry, so here is an answer to their problem – a diet on which you feel full, because high-fibre foods are so filling – and yet one that doesn't put on weight. In fact, the use of the word 'diet' in this context is strictly wrong. Whoever heard of a wild animal on a diet? Wild animals simply eat the food that's best for them, and so should we.

The last section of the book tells you how to live on unrefined foods and you'll notice at once that it's different from other slimming methods. It's a way of life and not a prohibitive, unnatural collection of rules. Once you get into it, you'll never look back.

Don't expect miracles though. The body's fat stores don't simply melt away overnight – you have to use up the energy they contain slowly. Going on to a high-fibre diet won't work wonders in the short term. But in the long term your high-fibre diet will pay off handsomely. It usually takes 10–20 years to get really fat; it will take a long time to get back to normal again.

One final word. There's no point only taking heed of part of the story and then complaining that it doesn't work. Some people claim that although they're taking bran morning, noon and night, they're still putting on weight. The trouble is they're not cutting out refined carbohydrates as well, and no responsible doctor would suggest that adding fibre to your diet will in itself work miracles in weight reduction. The answer must be a complete rethink of all the foods you eat, including the fatty ones. There's very little point in eating wholemeal bread if you smother it with an inch of jam or a lot of butter, or in eating high-fibre cereals and covering them with sugar. The beauty of the high-fibre method, as you'll see in the last section of the book, is that it's a 'thou shalt' and *not* a 'thou shalt not' diet. What more could you want?

9 Diabetes . . . sugar, the vice of all things nice

Diabetes is a disorder of body chemistry (metabolism) which produces a high blood sugar level, and sugar in the urine. The high blood sugar can cause problems in many different organs in the body.

As a disease, it's been known since ancient times. Indian physicians described it before the time of Christ, but it was the Greeks who gave it the name *diabetes* (Greek for a syphon) because they were impressed by the amount of urine passed by those suffering from it. In 1679 the term *mellitus* (honey-sweet) was added to describe the taste of the urine in diabetes.

For all this though, it wasn't until 1889 that it was found that removing a dog's pancreas made the dog diabetic. From then until 1921, when a team of medical scientists in Canada led by Banting and Best prepared an extract of dog's pancreas (insulin) capable of correcting diabetes, nothing much happened. Since the discovery of insulin in 1921, our knowledge of this strange and complex disease has grown – which is just as well, because so has the number of sufferers.

Diabetes was undoubtedly rare in past centuries. Galen, perhaps the most distinguished of ancient physicians, is said to have reported only two cases in 36 years of practice. Until this century it was still very uncommon, and men suffered from it more than women.

After 1923 it started to become much more common in women, and today it's right up among the top few killer diseases of the West. From being 27th on the causes of death list in 1900, that's quite a growth.

So here again we see a 'new' disease this century in the West. I say 'in the West' because numerous studies from all over the world show diabetes to be very rare in rural populations eating unrefined foods. It seems, however, that as rural people move into towns and take on our eating habits, they tend to become diabetic.

But just in case you think diabetes is a rare condition and so hardly worth considering – unless of course you've got it – just remember that there are probably well over 40 million diabetics in the world – the vast majority of them in the West. In Western Europe between 1 and 2 per cent of the population are known diabetics, and in the USA there are four million sufferers – nearly 2 per cent of the population. And for every known case there are probably four undiagnosed, walking around in the community! If this isn't enough, just bear in mind that diabetes is commonest in old people and that we have more elderly than ever before; and that good obstetric care means that babies of diabetic mothers who previously would have died now live, and you can see that we have a big and ever-growing diabetic problem in the West.

Most non-medical people imagine that because we can treat diabetes with insulin today, we have the disease beaten. Unfortunately, this is far from the truth. Certainly, insulin means that some diabetics (about one in five) are helped, but they are not *cured*. Although the patient's pancreas cannot make enough insulin, he doesn't stop being a diabetic when you inject him with it. He certainly lives longer than he otherwise would, but he still has a greater than average chance of dying prematurely, usually because of disease of the arteries.

Before we go any further and see how refined foods play an important part in causing diabetes, let's just see what diabetes is.

Every cell in the body needs energy to keep it alive. This energy comes from glucose, and the substance that controls how much glucose goes into the cells is insulin. After a meal, sugars and starches (the carbohydrates) are digested to produce glucose, which is then absorbed into the bloodstream to reach the whole body. Cells take up as much glucose as they need, and the excess is stored in the liver as a substance called *glycogen*. This is the body's store of glucose for when it's needed. If we didn't have this buffer store we'd need to be eating almost continuously so as to get enough energy to keep ourselves alive. When the liver stores are full of glycogen, the excess glucose is stored as fat in the body.

Except immediately following a meal, the level of glucose in the blood is fairly constant and is kept that way by a complex group of hormones. Should the liver's glycogen stores become exhausted, after a long fast for instance, the liver can actually manufacture new glucose from the body's fats and proteins. This is absolutely crucial because after oxygen, the body's greatest need is for glucose, or the cells will die.

Diabetics have too little effective insulin, so their cells can't use the glucose in the bloodstream. This leads to very high blood levels of glucose, which spill over into the urine. Normally of course the kidneys don't allow this valuable glucose to be wasted, but in diabetics they're simply overwhelmed by too much of it.

Unfortunately no one knows exactly what causes this lack of insulin, but several things are known. Most diabetics, contrary to popular belief, don't need insulin at all. About four out of five diabetics are of the so-called 'maturity-onset' type and these are very different from the 'insulin dependent' or 'juvenile' type.

The juvenile diabetic whose disease appears in childhood or adolescence has a relative lack of insulin in his body. It's possible that he may also produce abnormal insulin that the body's cells can't 'recognise', so resulting in the formation of antibodies to his insulin. The maturity-onset diabetic usually produces a fair amount of insulin or even too much on occasions, but there is still too little to go round all the cells in the body. And the reason why? Largely because he has too many cells – that is, he's obese.

So here we see one of the most serious results of obesity – a killer disease that can incapacitate the sufferer for years and yet is curable by one simple measure – slimming.

When we look back historically it's possible to parallel the incidence of obesity in almost any society with the level of diabetes. Obesity was rare in ancient Rome, Greece and Egypt – so was diabetes. The numbers of women dying from diabetes went down during both World Wars when rationing was in force and less food was consumed. Modern medical practice proves that dieting is the only treatment that 80 per cent of maturity-onset diabetics need. Take off their weight and their insulin can cope again. Almost all juvenile diabetics require insulin. Before we see how diabetes can be at least partly explained, and certainly helped by unrefined foods, let's look at one important predisposing factor – heredity.

Diabetes is certainly hereditary, but the exact mode of inheritance is as yet unknown. In juvenile-onset diabetes inheritance plays a major part, but in maturity-onset diabetes this is very much less important. Environmental factors determine the age of onset of diabetes. In certain highly susceptible people, diabetes will appear in childhood, but in the majority the disease doesn't become apparent until middle age. Probably as many as 10 per cent of the whole population of the United States has an inherited tendency to diabetes, but only a small proportion, about 8 per cent, will develop obvious or concealed signs of the disease if they reach 50–60 years of age. This is important when considering how fibre-free foods actually work in diabetes, because one of them, sugar, may well be the critical environmental factor that pushes a person with a diabetic tendency into a frank disease state.

But is it possible that fibre-free foods in general and sugar in particular actually cause diabetes? The short answer is that we don't know as yet, but it seems likely that sugar and perhaps even fat play a part.

As we've already seen in the obesity chapter, high-fibre foods tend to be naturally slimming, which must be helpful both in preventing and treating maturity-onset diabetes. Animal experiments back this up too. Mice, monkeys and sandrats, all of which rarely develop obesity or diabetes, can be made fat and diabetic by letting them feed freely on refined foods. In one experiment using mice, they all became normal again and regained normal blood sugar levels within a few days of switching back to a high-fibre diet.

This fits in very well with human studies during the period of food rationing in World War Two. During this time the consumption of sugar fell dramatically. This was also accompanied by a rise in the amount of fibre in the British diet because bread was less refined and contained more bran. The death rate from diabetes during the period 1941 to 1954 fell by 50–60 per cent while the nation was eating National Flour. The graph of diabetic deaths then started to pick up again from the early fifties as the fibre content of flour was decreased, and the nation's consumption of sugar and fat went up.

This wartime 'protective' effect of increasing fibre intake needs explaining, because experience from the rest of the world teaches us that it takes on average about twenty years for diabetes to appear in a community after it starts eating refined foods. So why was the change in diabetic deaths apparent so soon? During the last war what we saw was a fall in the level of fatal diabetes because the less refined diet kept it in check. That's not to say that there weren't just as many people 'at risk' of becoming diabetic, but simply that they didn't get overwhelmed with refined flour and sugar and so didn't suffer from the disease. It was simply a supply and overflow problem, with the increased wartime fibre intake and decreased sugar availability stemming the overflow.

Having said this though, it's important to remember that no humans have ever been cured of diabetes by cutting out sugar alone. Work currently under way in California has shown that 'cures' or permanent remissions in diabetes can be achieved by increasing an individual's intake of unrefined cereals, cutting out sugar completely and reducing fat intake. This fits in well with wartime evidence, which shows that in 1940 when sugar consumption decreased by 20 per cent in the UK, fats by 8 per cent and there was *no change* in dietary fibre intake, death rates from diabetes *rose*. But in 1941 when sugar consumption fell by 25 per cent, fats by 12 per cent and *there was a rise* in dietary fibre intake of 50 per cent, death rates from diabetes *fell*.

But if middle-age diabetes is largely an obesity-orientated problem and is fairly straightforward to treat, the juvenile or insulin-dependent kind certainly isn't. This more troublesome type of diabetes is caused, as we've seen, by a relative lack of insulin production. No one knows why this should occur and there are probably many factors. Some experts would maintain that in certain susceptible people unrefined starches and sugar somehow put demands on the pancreas with which it can't cope. When we eat unrefined foods we take our carbohydrates in a relatively 'dilute' form. The amounts of fibre bound up with starches and sugars also mean that they are more slowly digested and probably more slowly absorbed. This in turn prevents big surges of sugar from being absorbed into the bloodstream after each meal. Also, by insuring that the blood sugar level doesn't fluctuate wildly, the strains on the pancreas to provide a balancing amount of insulin are bound to be less. One researcher reported his dramatic findings on this to the seventh Congress of the International Diabetic Federation in 1971. He found that pure sugar consumption produced gigantic rises in blood sugar compared with the gentle waves produced by eating the same number of calories in the form of apples and potatoes. Even peeling the potatoes (and so refining them) made a noticeable difference to the blood sugar curve.

So it's quite possible that these stresses of glucose load, and the consequent insulin production, may quite quickly so damage the pancreas's ability to produce more insulin that in some people it shuts down completely.

Some doctors now think that the juvenile type of diabetes is caused by a similar reaction to sugar itself. It's amazing just how early in life we are assaulted by sugar. In many maternity units a newborn baby is given sugar water as soon as it's born. Many mothers add sugar to milk feeds because they think the child will like them better, to stop constipation, or to give the baby 'more energy'.

It is true that some baby milks don't have enough calories without additional sugar, but the instructions will always spell this out carefully. Babies won't get constipated if they have enough fluid, and boiled water is better than anything when it comes to fluid replacement. Adding sugar as an anti-constipating substance simply compounds the felony of most modern mothers – overfeeding. As was pointed out in the chapter on obesity, the first few weeks or months of a baby's life are critical in conditioning it to refined carbohydrate intake. It's an indictment of modern society that most babies are addicted to carbohydrates from their earliest days – an addiction for which they pay very dearly in later life.

Undoubtedly, the enormous consumption of highly refined foods has a lot to do with diabetes at all ages but it's probably fair to say that it's only one factor, albeit a major one, in the production of this disabling and killing disease.

10 Gallstones . . . rocks for ages, made by me

The gallbladder is a strange organ. Man has one but horses, rats and birds don't – the giraffe sometimes does and sometimes doesn't. Most of us know someone who's had gallstones or jaundice, the two most common results of gallbladder disease.

As an organ the gallbladder is rather unimpressive. It's a small, pear-shaped sac about two-and-a-half inches long, lying beneath the liver immediately underneath the right rib cage. It stores and concentrates bile which is constantly produced by the liver. It then ejects the bile into the duodenum after meals. Bile itself is a greeny-yellow fluid made up of two main substances, bile salts and bile pigments. Bile salts come from cholesterol, of which more later, and bile pigments have to do with the normal breakdown of red blood cells.

Bile salts play a vital role in fat digestion. They reduce the size of fat globules in our food by a sort of detergent action, making the fats into a milky liquid composed of very fine particles. This action of bile salts is rather like the mixing of oil and vinegar for a salad dressing, and anyone who's done this will know how difficult it is to break up the oil (fat) into tiny particles. The salts then help the fats we eat to be absorbed through the wall of the small intestine. Apart from this function in fat digestion, they're also essential in vitamin absorption – so obviously they're very valuable body substances.

So valuable are the bile salts that the body tends to conserve them. When they're re-absorbed from the bowel they get transported back to the liver and resecreted into the bile. It's been calculated that from their starting point as a product of cholesterol, bile salts recirculate as many as 18 times before being finally passed out of the body in the stools.

I've explained all this at some length because bile salts play a big part in our modern views on gallstones, and seem to be especially involved in gallstone formation in those of us eating refined diets. But first let's look at the size of the gallstone problem.

It's difficult to know just how common gallstones are because you can have them for years and never know, but it's generally accepted that by the age of 70 at least 30 per cent of women and 15 per cent of men will have them.

As gallbladder disease in the Western world is almost entirely due to gallstones, it's well worth knowing how they form so that we can try and prevent them. To all intents and purposes Western gallstones are made of cholesterol: UK, American and Swedish stones are composed of 60, 74 and 88 per cent cholesterol respectively. On the other hand, few people on unrefined diets in Africa and Asia ever get gallstones, and when they do they're usually made of bile pigments and not cholesterol.

The operation for the removal of the gallbladder is the commonest elective (non-urgent) abdominal operation in the Western world, about a million gallbladders being removed every year. It's a sobering fact that more money is spent on removing gallbladders in the USA than is spent on all medical services in the continent of Africa. But then gallstones are very common in the West. More than a third of a million gallbladders are taken out in the USA every year alone, and American women have more gallbladders removed than appendices.

As all the latest theories on gallstones revolve around the much maligned substance cholesterol, and because cholesterol crops up in several other chapters, let's take a look at this remarkable body substance.

Cholesterol first came before the public eye when the arguments over saturated and unsaturated fats were in full swing. These fats, and cholesterol in particular, came in for a lot of criticism because they were thought to be instrumental in blocking the arteries in heart disease. But whether or not cholesterol is the ogre of this particular story (see chapter eleven), it's far from a nuisance to the body – it's an essential part of its chemistry.

Cholesterol belongs to the group of fatty substances in the body called lipids. Cholesterol in the superficial layers of the skin is turned into Vitamin D by sunlight, and is also the basic building block for many of the body's hormones. It is produced throughout the body, except perhaps by the nerve cells, but in largest amounts by the liver, skin and bowel walls, which together produce about 98 per cent of the body's supply. Of course we can also get cholesterol by eating it in foods such as eggs, meat, cheese, milk, cream, ice cream, chocolate and nuts, but the average person produces more than he eats.

Someone of average weight (about 150 lb) will have about 60 g of cholesterol in his body, of which 1 g a day is lost and replaced. But because he's producing about 800 mg himself and taking in yet more from his food, he's always well into 'credit' with his cholesterol bank. Even though some of this excess is made into bile salts there is still an excess of cholesterol, which may have serious consequences in heart disease as we shall see, but for the moment let's stay with gallstones.

A fat person who's about 30 per cent overweight produces 75 per cent more cholesterol than he needs – in fact an obese person's liver may put out twice as much cholesterol in a day as that of the average lean person. Fat people produce more cholesterol in their livers because of the excess calories they take in, a fact well proven by laboratory experiments. Yet this is not because they absorb more cholesterol from their fatty and fattening food, but because the fattening diet persuades their livers to make more cholesterol. In fact there seems to be a sophisticated balancing mechanism in healthy people which ensures that if the intestine is absorbing more cholesterol than usual from food, the liver will produce less. But all this knowledge is very new.

Gallstones were probably rare, even in the West, until this century, but we've already seen how difficult it is to assess the incidence of a disease like this that doesn't necessarily produce symptoms. Post-mortem studies, a major source of present-day information, weren't carried out on large enough numbers of people until this century. Famous medical writers of the past hardly mention gallstones, but most experts seem to agree that the richer classes must have had them. Evidence to support this theory comes from such finds as a Chinese mummy dating back to 2000 BC which was recently found to have them. But as far as we can tell, gallstones weren't at all common, let alone of the epidemic proportions they are today, until this century at least, and even then probably not until as recently as 1945.

So, assuming as we must that there's a linking factor between the rich people in the past and the majority of Western people today, and that poor non-Westerners both historically and today seem to be protected somehow from gallstones, let's look at some contemporary evidence.

1 Gallstones used to be seen in rich people – now they're seen in all classes.
2 They used to be a disease of middle age – now they're found at all ages. In Sweden, operations for the removal of gallstones in children are not at all uncommon.
3 This spread through the ages is paralleled by a spread in obesity.
4 As populations change from eating high-fibre diets to refined diets, their level of gallstones goes up dramatically. This change in diet often goes with a change from rural to urban living. A famous surgeon working in rural Africa for 17 years operated on only two patients with gallstones, and one of those was a queen.

The only single factor that links all these things is the urbanisation of the people concerned and their consumption of refined foods. Enormous rises in the occurrence of gallstones have now been reported in the Japanese, Eskimos, Africans and American negroes as they become urbanised and eat our Western food.

So how does a refined diet cause gallstones? Probably in two main ways.

The first of these involves cholesterol. We've seen already just how easy it is to eat refined foods and so to take in large numbers of calories. Research now shows that when we take in large slugs of energy the liver produces more cholesterol. This is especially true, as we've seen, in fat people. Studies on known gallstone patients also show that they take in more calories than control patients. When a graph is drawn of obesity since 1945 against the incidence of gallstones, the parallel is obvious between the numbers of people suffering from obesity and the numbers of cases of gallstones; and so is the decreasing age of onset of both obesity and stones.

Further, obese middle-aged diabetics (the commonest of diabetics) have more gallstones than normal people, and gallstone patients themselves are more likely to be diabetic. The Pima Indians are exceedingly obese and have the highest level of diabetes and gallstones in the world.

Gallstones seem to be linked inextricably with obesity and diabetes, themselves both diseases of overconsumption; so as we know that fat people produce more cholesterol and cholesterol is the main source of gallstones, we seem to be getting closer to an answer.

Let's take a look at animal experiments to produce gallstones, because in animals it's possible to control all the food factors more easily than in man. In different groups of animals fed on all sorts of diets in numerous experiments all over the world, there was only one sure way of producing gallstones ... by giving them low-fibre, highly refined foods. On highly refined foods the bile becomes oversaturated with cholesterol and so it is more likely that stones will precipitate out. Not only does the gallbladder level of cholesterol go up in people on highly refined diets, but their total amount of bile salts (which normally hold cholesterol in solution) goes down. Why should this be?

As yet research is at an early stage, but it has shown that refined diets somehow reduces the amount of bile salts made by the liver. This tends to lead to stone formation. Recent experiments involving the feeding of certain bile salts to patients with stones, show that the stones are actually dissolved – probably because cholesterol secretion is reduced.

These bile salts are breakdown products of cholesterol in the liver, and are composed of three substances – deoxycholate (20 per cent), chenodeoxycholate (35–40 per cent) and cholate (40–45 per cent).

Deoxycholate is normally absorbed in the colon and re-used

by the body. Because the stools in people on refined foods are so small and hard, and take so long to pass through the colon, there's more time for deoxycholate (usually only partly absorbed) to be absorbed in greater quantities. The resulting high blood level of deoxycholate suppresses the formation of chenodeoxycholate in the liver. This is bad because chenodeoxycholate is nature's own chemical way of preventing gallstones before they start. When there is little chenodeoxycholate a stone can form and grow quickly in the saturated, cholesterol-rich bile, which is also caused by refined foods.

So efficient is this substance (chenodeoxycholate) in dissolving gallstones that it has been purified and is now available commercially. It is being used on certain gallstone patients instead of an operation, but it will unfortunately dissolve only stones rich in cholesterol, and it only works if the gallbladder is still functioning. As the symptoms of gallstones tend to be so vague, the condition is often diagnosed late and the gallbladder is in a poor state by this stage or even not working at all. If it is working well, even quite large stones (up to half an inch across) can be dissolved within six months to two years using chenodeoxycholate by mouth.

Dr K. Heaton, working in Bristol, has pieced together all these complex factors of body chemistry, geography, history and diet and devised a simple set of experiments to test his hypothesis that gallstones are in fact caused by consumption of refined, low-residue foods. He fed bran to volunteers and found that deoxycholate was reduced by 30 per cent and that chenodeoxycholate was increased. He also found that bran-treated patients produced bile less rich in cholesterol. This was followed by a study in which women with gallstones were fed bran – their bile cholesterol fell by 30 per cent.

So it's clear from this and other available evidence that eating highly refined foods increases the likelihood of getting gallstones.

Dr Cleave agrees with Heaton that sugar too has an important part to play in the formation of gallstones, but for different reasons. Dr Heaton maintains that sugar is harmful because it causes overnutrition and so the growth of gallstones.

Dr Cleave suggests that the excess sugar in a Western refined diet encourages the bacteria normally present in the bowel (and in the gallbladder) to reproduce more vigorously than normal, and that the larger numbers of these bacteria found in people on refined diets is the reason why cholesterol forms stones in the first place. After all, not everyone with a high gallbladder level of cholesterol makes stones, so these bacteria may well be the initiating factor. But it must be stressed that the triggering of gallstone formation can only occur when the bile is super-saturated with cholesterol – which therefore must be the basic abnormality.

If this bacterial theory were true it would nicely bridge the gap between the old theory that gallstones were formed because of large numbers of bacteria in the gallbladder, and the newer cholesterol theory. It's probable though that neither too many bacteria nor too much cholesterol alone will produce stones, but that a combination of the two is necessary. As we've seen, they're both closely linked to the eating of refined foods, so we know where the solution must lie.

11 Coronaries . . . the way to a man's heart

Coronary artery disease, the cause of heart attacks, claims the lives of one in three men in the Western world. Such is the enormity of the problem that some experts have called it 'The greatest epidemic ever known to man.'

Man has had to cope with epidemics before in his history, as we saw in chapter two, but this one's different – it cuts down men in their prime, at a time when their commitments to their families and work are greatest. So serious is this epidemic that researchers the world over have been looking for a cure for more than 30 years, with no real success. But we can't give up – heart attacks are affecting younger men and are now affecting women too. In fact, the latest figures show that heart attacks are now more efficient than ever at killing us off. The actual mortality from heart disease has increased more than threefold in the last 15 years.

However emotive a subject cancer may be, coronary heart disease claims three times more victims than all forms of cancer put together – so an answer has to be found.

The amazing thing is that until about 1920 heart attacks, and the condition called *angina pectoris* which often precedes them, were very uncommon in the West. Certainly, doctors knew about angina centuries ago. The famous physician Heberden wrote his classical description as long ago as 1768. After all, this tight, gripping pain like a constricting band around the chest is so characteristic it would have been hard to miss; yet physicians like Heberden only came across it rarely.

Remember too, that we're talking about an era when post-mortem studies were very commonly performed, so had coronary heart disease been at all commonplace, the doctors of the day would have recorded it. The changes in the heart muscle are often plain to see even to the naked, untrained eye.

In 1893–4 the distinguished Canadian doctor Sir William Osler, an expert of considerable renown, reported seeing only five cases of angina in 8860 medical patients at his hospital. Only 13 years later he was able to document 268 cases in detail.

All the evidence shows that between 1880 and 1904 the death rate from coronary artery disease was constant at about 22 per million of the population of the UK. By 1915 the level had reached 35 per million; by 1925 47 per million; and by 1930, 148 per million – a tremendous increase. But it wasn't until nearly 1930 that really accurate diagnosis became the norm when, because of electrocardiographic (ECG) evidence, doctors could ascertain the trouble with the heart more clearly. This meant that some people who would otherwise have died from a 'cause unknown' could now be seen to have underlying heart disease diagnosed from the ECG before death.

By 1931 the death rate from coronary heart disease, was 166 per million and by 1969 it had soared to 2856 per million. So in 90 years its incidence had risen 142-fold. Because of better diagnosis? Unlikely.

This is a true epidemic which has its roots somewhere in the 1880–1890s and is continuing unabated to the present day.

Yet in all the developing and rural countries of the world this epidemic has *not* struck. Coronary artery disease is rare in rural Africa and Asia, and studies with the best methods known to modern medicine can find only scant evidence of this number-one Western killer in these communities.

Except in the cities that is, when people take on our Western way of life. Doctors studying certain urbanised groups in Indian cities now find exactly the same level of ECG abnormalities suggestive of coronary artery disease as can be found in American or European cities. Couple this with the fact that people of Japanese and Negro stock living in the USA have the same level of heart disease as have their white compatriots, and you'll see that it's not simply a matter of genetics either.

Heart disease is caused by something in our environment in the West, and it is killing off our men at an alarming rate. If

you're over 40 you have a 50–50 chance of having a heart attack
before you're 65. A sobering thought. If you should get a heart
attack, you've got a 30-per cent chance of dying within the first
24 hours. If you get over the first few weeks, you've still only
five to seven years to look forward to on average. In Britain
today, the average doctor lives long enough to collect six
months of his pension – heart attacks claim most of the rest.

Before we go on to look at what causes heart attacks, let's see
what the heart is and how it works.

Quite simply the heart is a hollow, muscular chamber about
the size of your fist. It contracts spontaneously 70 times a
minute every minute of our lives. That's over 100,000 beats a
day for 70 years or 2575 million beats in a lifetime! Yet it never
stops for rest and never gets serviced! The heart *mustn't* stop
because if it were to, the blood supplying the rest of the body
with its vital oxygen and energy would stop flowing, so leading
to death of the body's tissues. If the heart stops for more than
two minutes, irreparable damage is done to the delicate brain
cells.

All the heart asks for in return for this lifelong service is
plenty of oxygen-rich blood containing the nutrients it needs to
keep pumping. The blood supply to the heart comes through
two small arteries – the coronary arteries. These encircle the
heart and branch to supply all its parts. The trouble with the
coronary arteries is that if they get blocked the results are immediately felt and the damage produced is serious. In many
other parts of the body small arteries can be shut off without
much damage – other arteries in the area enlarge and supply the
blood-starved part, so all is well. In the heart, every little
branch of the coronary arteries is important, so the slightest
blockage results in death of the part of the heart muscle supplied by that branch.

Heart muscle, unlike some other tissues in the body, once
dead, stays dead. If a large part of a coronary artery becomes
blocked, the heart stops working properly because so much of
its muscle is without essential oxygen and the whole heart
ceases to pump efficiently. This is called heart failure. It sets up
a vicious circle, because if the heart isn't pumping blood

around to the lungs to pick up more oxygen, then it obviously can't be getting enough oxygen itself. Eventually, the whole heart becomes so starved of oxygen that the nervous connections that keep the heartbeats going are unable to function and the heart dies.

Why, you may ask, should the coronary arteries become blocked in the first place? The answer is not simple. As we in the Western world age, our arteries become impregnated with a thick porridge-like substance called *atheroma*. This tends to involve the large arteries (such as the aorta) and the medium-sized ones (like the coronaries). This fatty substance can be seen in the arterial walls of children undergoing post-mortem examination after car accidents for instance, and was found to be almost universal in the arteries of young US soldiers killed in Vietnam and Korea.

As the arterial walls thicken with these fatty deposits, scar tissue appears in them, healthy tissue is destroyed and a small haemorrhage occurs under the thin lining of the wall. This results in a slow narrowing of the canal rather like the furring up of pipes in a hard-water area. Slowly, the channel becomes so narrow that the amount of blood getting through is severely restricted.

This may not matter while the person's heart is resting, but as soon as he exerts himself, the extra oxygen needed by the heart simply can't get there because the arteries are so obstructed. Waste products build up in the muscle and can't get away. The pain that these waste products produce is called *angina*.

The other problem with atheroma is that it can cause a sudden block in an artery. The roughened, fatty areas of arterial lining are especially likely to form small blood clots which may shut off the canal at that point or be washed downstream into a narrower artery which becomes blocked off entirely.

Just what causes atheroma is not known, but because it contains lots of fatty material and especially cholesterol, doctors have tended to think that cholesterol is to blame. This may not be the whole truth, as we shall see.

So what causes heart attacks? Why do some people with just as much atheroma as others never get them?

The simple answer is, we don't know but we're getting on to the track. When any disease seems to be related or linked to several variables, doctors call it multifactorial. This is a word meaning that they haven't yet decided which of all the seemingly linked facts actually causes the disease. There's no point saying (as indeed many doctors did) that poor living conditions cause tuberculosis. The TB bacillus causes it, and poor housing helps to create the right environment for the bacilli to get a hold.

It's the same with heart disease. So frantic has the search been for possible causes that the list of suspects grows yearly. It now includes fats, smoking, stress, lack of exercise, drinking soft water, high blood pressure, obesity, diabetes, genetic factors and many more. What is far more likely in my opinion is that there is an underlying *cause per se* and that some of these other things help to aggravate the situation in certain susceptible people.

Because very convincing evidence is often put forward to support these ideas, it's worth just looking at some of them to see why they don't hold water in the light of the high fibre story.

The consumption of fat has always been top of the list of horrors in the war against heart disease. For many years we've been told that too much fat silts up our arteries. The Western world has been inundated with cholesterol-free foods and polyunsaturated fats. Because cholesterol was found to be the main fat present in atheromatous arteries it was assumed that we were eating too much of it and that it was being deposited in our blood vessels. This theory is now losing ground in the eyes of the experts for many reasons. For a start, the level of cholesterol in the blood (and hence one presumes in the arterial walls) doesn't necessarily bear a close relation to the level of heart disease.

Certainly, statistics can be drawn up to show that with more than a certain level of cholesterol in the blood a person is more likely to have a heart attack. The interesting thing is that this 'certain level' varies from country to country – and by quite a lot. In the USA a level of more than 265 mg/100 ml of blood is considered undesirable; in Norway, 270 mg/100 ml; in Italy 202 mg/100 ml and India 195 mg/100 ml. Some authorities don't even worry until the level reaches the 300 mark. So where does this leave us? Confused, because certain groups of Africans in whom coronary artery disease is almost unknown, have the same cholesterol levels as we do in the West.

For years we've been taught to think of saturated (animal) fat as being bad for us because it silts up our arteries. Margarines and spreads made from plant oils (sunflower or cotton seed usually) are relatively new products. These plant seed oils are called polyunsaturated fats and are said to be less harmful than animal fats. Some experts even claim they have a positive value in their own right in heart disease. But this obsession with fat being so unhealthy or even the cause of heart disease seems unnecessary. Man has been eating fats for centuries. Neolithic man had both animals and milk, and 1500 years before Moses the Bible tells us of Jehovah's instruction to his people to eat 'butter of kine, and milk of sheep, with fat of lambs'.

On the contrary, eating seed oils is new and somewhat contrived, because over the centuries man has become adapted to eating animal fat and certainly ought to be able to cope with it. The Masai and Eskimos, great meat-, milk- and fat-eaters, do not have our epidemic of heart disease, and a study of Bulgarian peasants living almost exclusively on milk and dairy produce found that they were extremely long lived.

On top of this, the great increase in fat consumption in the West took place in the 1930s – ten years after the start of the heart disease epidemic. So it hardly looks as though fat is the main cause.

But if the Masai, Eskimos and other peoples of the world have managed to adapt to eating fat, why haven't we? Could it be that we've lost something from our diet that protects us from the dangers of fat over-consumption?

An interesting study of Indian railway sweepers found that heart disease was seven times more common in the South of India than in the North. In the South, the diet consisted mostly of refined rice and only three-and-a-half per cent of daily calories were taken as fat (as polyunsaturated seed oils mostly). In the North, the diet was unrefined wheat and maize with 23 per cent of calories eaten as saturated animal fats. Polyunsaturated fats made up 45 per cent of the fats in the South but only 2 per cent in the North, and even so coronary artery disease was much commoner in the South.

Clearly, the fat saga is going to be with us for some time yet but the problem with a low-fat diet, even if it should be found helpful, is that it's so unpalatable. Avoiding fat and all the foods containing cholesterol (see chapter ten, on gallstones) makes the diet almost inedible to most people. There may well be an alternative.

Now to some other suspects. Cigarette smoking is undoubtedly harmful and causes lung cancer. It must be seen as only an aggravating factor though in heart disease, because so many people who have never smoked still die of heart disease. The nicotine in cigarettes may well cause small branches of the coronary arteries to contract, so precipitating a heart attack, and for this reason cigarettes are to be avoided from the heart's point of view. And smoking definitely increases your chances of having a heart attack (smokers have three times the likelihood of dying from heart disease as do non-smokers). But almost certainly it doesn't cause them.

The part played by smoking in aggravating heart disease however shouldn't be underestimated. Doctors in the UK took the lead in the anti-smoking campaign and cut down more effectively than their patients. It's been estimated that the number of doctors' lives saved each year as a result, is the same as the output of an average medical school. Well worth the effort!

Lack of exercise is also thought by many to be one of the causes of heart disease. Supporters of this theory point to the active, physically athletic Africans and Asians, and assume that this is the reason that they are free from the scourge of heart disease. Certainly, too little exercise combined with too much of our Western food will make people fat, which then increases the risk of heart disease. But exercise itself seems to be less important than other things in its prevention. Finnish lumber-jacks, hardly inactive, have the highest level of coronary heart disease in the world.

Stress is often said to be the biggest cause of heart disease. The advocates of this theory cite the absence of heart disease in the developing countries as clear evidence that stress is responsible for our heart problems in the West. But this is arrogance indeed. To suggest that we in the West are 'stressed' and that the rest of the world has an easy time of it, is not only chauvinistic but frankly wrong.

The stresses of life in an African or Asian rural community are very considerable. We in the West are pampered by comparison. We rarely have to concern ourselves with shelter, extremes of temperature, scavenging for food, climatic excesses, endless infections, high childhood mortality, enormous birthrates, poor transport, famine or drought. Throughout his evolution man has had to contend with stress and overcome it. There have been no signs of wartime epidemics of heart disease this century, and war is clearly a time when both civilian and fighting populations are subjected to real stress for year after year. On the contrary, during these crises all over Europe and even inside towns under siege, the amount of heart disease fell. This may be linked to an increase in the amount of un-refined foods consumed during wartime rationing.

An American, Dr Rahe, has related the pattern of certain events in people's lives to their major illnesses, especially heart attacks. The score on his table corresponded to the likelihood that the patient would have a heart attack, and he found that the crises in the subject's life usually occurred several years before the heart attack, suggesting that there might be a cause-and-effect relationship. It is certainly reasonable to suppose that worry over long periods can induce physical ill health; but we cannot assume that the things we find stressful are of no importance to the other two-thirds of the world's population that *don't* get heart disease.

After all, of the top twenty items in Dr Rahe's table, at least 18 must be judged as stressful to a rural African or Indian as they are to us. Add to these all the extra stresses that these people have, and it's possible to argue that stress might even prevent heart attacks! Another interesting fact is that Africans who smoke, are overweight, have high blood pressure or diabetes, *don't* have an increased risk of getting heart disease as we do. Could it be that in spite of all the aggravating factors being present, they are protected in some way? Until they go into the cities and take on our way of life, that is.

The answer seems to be 'yes'. Something protects them and that something seems to be dietary fibre. So how does it work?

Let's start by looking at fats. As we've seen, an excess of cholesterol has been thought to be dangerous. So until we know what in fact causes atheroma, it would seem sensible to try and keep the cholesterol level in our blood down to levels at which heart attacks are rare. The difficulty we come across at once is that authorities disagree as to what this 'normal' level should be. Add to this the fact that some communities with blood-cholesterol levels as high as ours in the West never get coronary heart disease, and the problem becomes even more complicated.

Simply cutting down on the intake of cholesterol as milk, eggs, cream and butter may not be the answer, because the body continues to make its own cholesterol and may even step up production if intake is reduced.

Reducing saturated animal fat intake is probably worthwhile, although just how important this is, is not yet clear. Part of the confusion arises because the way the body handles fats, including cholesterol, seems to alter according to the amount of fibre in the diet.

Numerous experiments have shown that blood cholesterol levels fall when people eat high-fibre foods, but the fall is often only temporary. Third- and fourth-generation Italians in the USA eating their traditional food (rich in fibre) have less coronary heart disease than their American compatriots, although they both eat the same amount of fat. A basic USA hospital diet might contain 4·0 g of fibre per day, while a Southern Italian one has 18·8 g per day.

A fascinating study in Ireland also shows how fibre can protect against heart disease. In Irish men aged between 45 and 64, 29 per cent of all deaths are due to coronary artery disease.

This figure compares with 42 per cent of second-generation Irish living in Massachusetts. Autopsy studies show that atheroma occurs much later and less severely in the Irish compared with the Americans.

In this particular study, 1154 age-matched pairs of Irish brothers who both grew up in Ireland were followed up after one brother had emigrated to the USA. On the ECG evidence of heart disease, the Irish brothers had 2·1 per cent abnormal traces compared with the Americans' 4 per cent. The Irish brothers actually ate *more* animal fat, but had similar serum cholesterol levels. All other variables such as smoking, sugar, protein and cholesterol intake were the same for both groups, as were their blood pressures.

The main dietary difference was the amount of refined carbohydrate that each group ate. The Irish ate lots of potatoes (rich in fibre) and consumed 6·4 g of fibre per day on average. The American brothers only ate 3·6 g per day of fibre, mostly as fruit and vegetables. So the Irish men ate 78 per cent more fibre than their American brothers who got 90 per cent more heart disease.

Other research shows that it's not only how much fibre you take but how you take it that matters. For instance, blood cholesterol levels in animals are reduced more by eating intact rice than by eating refined rice to which the bran has been restored. In fact, this remained true even if the amount of fibre added was twice the original amount in the rice. Small amounts of fibre, taken as bran, probably don't alter blood cholesterol levels very much – you have to eat enormous amounts of fibre to have any meaningful effect. What we do know is that the absorption of cholesterol from the intestine is reduced in people eating high-fibre diets.

But there are other fats in the blood – the triglycerides – which may be more important in heart disease. This fraction of the blood fats has been known for years, but work on it hasn't progressed as far as that on cholesterol partly because triglyceride levels in the blood are so difficult to measure. Many diabetics and obese people have high blood triglycerides, and these very people also tend to get more coronary artery disease.

In the Western world, all the blood fats rise from childhood until the age of from 50 to 59 years. We assume that this is normal, although other communities don't show the rise in triglycerides that we do. A trial in Sweden followed 3168 men for nine years, and measured their cholesterol and triglyceride levels, relating them to the incidence of heart disease. The research found that the triglyceride levels were a much better risk indicator than were cholesterol levels. Work in America supports this by showing that heart attack survivors had triglyceride levels three times normal, and that more had high triglycerides than high cholesterols. So perhaps the days of worrying unduly about cholesterol are numbered.

The interesting thing about triglycerides is that their levels are influenced by our diet. Out of 16 people who were fed refined carbohydrate in one particular study, 15 showed an increase in triglycerides in their blood. Other research seems to prove that dietary fibre acts, in this context, by lowering blood triglycerides rather than by affecting cholesterol. The best experiment that supports this was done with 28 Cistercian Trappist monks. All the monks were asked to give up their normal diet of wholemeal bread. One half was given bran biscuits and the other half white bread. After 12 weeks, their cholesterol levels were not very different but the triglyceride levels were significantly reduced, especially in the under forties, in those on the bran biscuits.

By now you may be forgiven for thinking that the heart disease picture is somewhat confused. This is because heart disease is such an emotive and widely-researched subject that worldwide evidence is somewhat fragmentary. But we can say with some certainty that high-fibre diets seem to alter the body's chemistry towards that associated with a low incidence of heart disease. This in itself cannot be bad.

Heart attacks arise because of small blood clots in coronary arteries, as we've seen, so we can't leave the subject until we see how fibre might effect blood clotting. It's well known that high-fat diets tend to increase the coagulability of the blood. A study on a group of elderly Danes proved that when taken off fat they produced fewer clots in their bodies than before. But work on fibre and clotting is in its early days. Experiments on rats suggest that eating fibre protects them against clotting, and experiments on the speed at which the body breaks up clots once formed (a natural and continuous process) show that rural Africans break them up much quicker than Westerners living in the same area. This could of course also be linked to the amount of fat in their respective diets.

In the West we seem to have blood which clots peculiarly easily. Autopsies on 1427 Ugandans found that only 2·4 per cent of them had blood clots anywhere; but in a similar group of Americans, 52 per cent had clots. The answer to this difference may well lie, of all places, in the bacterial content of our large bowels. Some of these bacteria produce Vitamin K, a vital element in normal blood clotting. It's too early yet to say whether the change in colonic bacteria that occurs on low-fibre diets makes a difference in Vitamin K production and so to blood clotting, but work is well under way on this problem.

Arguments on blood fats and blood clotting will probably go on for years, but whatever the outcome, this we can say. High-fibre foods will tend to reduce the amount of heart disease, by reducing the number of people suffering from obesity and diabetes in the societies where heart disease is so common. It's been said that the greatest thing that's wrong with our food in the West is that there's too much of it. I would suggest that we eat the wrong kind of food. We've seen how obesity and diabetes can be remedied by a high-fibre diet, and since both of these can predispose towards heart attacks, we're well on the way to doing something really practical.

While we're talking about other fibre-linked diseases, it's interesting to note that diverticular disease of the colon (about as different from heart attacks as you can get!) emerged at the same time as coronary heart disease – in the 1920s. The two diseases are also found in parallel throughout the Western world as fibre is removed from the diet. As we now believe that diverticular disease is definitely caused by a lack of fibre in the diet, it would seem reasonable to wonder whether coronary artery disease might not also be linked to fibre lack. The simultaneous emergence of these two very different diseases seems too much of a coincidence to be ignored. Studies have now shown that the two diseases occur more commonly in an individual than you would expect statistically. One Australian study of 200 autopsies found that atheroma was much more common in people with severe diverticular disease than in those with very little of the disease.

What's needed now is a long-term trial with matched populations on high- and low-fibre diets, all other variables being kept the same. Unfortunately, trials like this are extremely difficult to mount and with the 'incubation period' of coronary heart disease set at about 20 years after the start of low-fibre feeding, it's going to be a 25-year study at least.

In the meantime, it's probably reasonable to reduce your saturated animal fat intake slightly by cutting the fat off meat and drinking skimmed milk, in addition to eating a high-fibre diet. It certainly can't harm you and might help reduce the odds in the Russian roulette of heart disease.

Results from a dietary trial during 1975 in California have yet to be confirmed but could open a new chapter in the treatment of arterial disease. Nearly 40 patients suffering from severe atheromatous disease of the arteries of the legs were divided into two groups. One ate US diets and received the latest medical treatment. They showed little improvement at the end of six months. The other group ate mostly unrefined starchy food (rich in fibre), very little fat and no sugar or salt.

They showed very great improvement. Three patients who had previously suffered from angina ceased to have attacks: and of 13 diabetics 11 were so improved that they required no treatment.

12 Bowel disease . . . the real pressures of the Western world

Have you ever thought that diseases as different as appendicitis, constipation, colon disease, varicose veins and piles could be caused by a common factor? I'm sure you haven't, because most doctors didn't themselves link these apparently very different diseases until very recently. Today, we can see how they fit together. A lack of dietary fibre has been incriminated as the single factor common to them all. Fortunately, we can do something about this very easily and very safely.

In fact, all these conditions are caused by 'pressure' of one kind or another in various parts of the body and so have been called 'pressure diseases' for short. In order to understand how fibre relieves pressure in organs as different as the appendix and the veins of the legs, we need to take a closer look at how fibre works in our intestine.

When food is eaten it is subjected to a myriad of chemical breakdown processes. We saw this in the chapter on obesity. Once our food reaches the end of its 23-feet journey through the small intestine it arrives in the large bowel or colon, where it is held awaiting disposal. What we haven't looked at is how long all this takes and why the speed at which the bowel propels food along is so important. The time that food and its residue take to be passed from mouth to anus is called the *transit time*.

As long ago as the beginning of this century research workers were wondering whether the speed of food transit through the body had any beneficial or any harmful effects. These early experimenters gave themselves and their subjects simple things like millet seeds to eat and then timed the interval until they appeared in the stools. As early as 1909 a red marker dye in gelatine capsules was used as a timing marker. Soon barium –

the radio-opaque substance given as a 'barium meal' so that the digestive tract will show up on X-rays – was being used as a marker. In the early 1950s, two leading nutritionists used white and wholemeal bread spread with barium on groups of subjects so that they could see how quickly each type of bread was digested and moved through the gut.

Slowly a picture was built up of the time for normal food, as eaten in the West, to pass through the bowel. Studies with barium showed that in over half the patients there was still some barium left in the bowel after 48 hours; in a quarter, *all* the barium was still in the bowel after 72 hours; and in one third of them there was still barium in the bowel after *five days*. Just contrast this with a similar study among rural Zulus, which showed that all of them had passed all the barium within 48 hours and you can see why the subject of transit times has aroused so much interest.

This interest in transit times has increased over the last few years because it has been realised that the diseases of the West are common only in populations whose transit times are long. By contrast, those people that have short transit times seldom suffer from our Western diseases. So, suddenly, the speed at which food passes through our bowels has taken on a new importance.

Recent experiments using plastic pellets show even more unexpected things about our bowels and the way they work. Because these pellets (about the size of a rice grain) are so easily dispersed in the bowel after being swallowed they show how food flows through the muscular tube which is our intestine. The plastic of which the pellets are made is impregnated with barium so that they can be seen on an X-ray at every stage of their passage through the intestine. With modern ciné X-rays it's even possible from such studies to see how food 'streams' in the bowel, forming eddy-currents and backwaters just like other liquids flowing in tubes.

Studies with these pellets have shown that in most people the time that food takes to reach the colon is fairly constant, and that the majority of the 25 pellets of the standard dose swallowed get to the large bowel all together. In the colon, however, the fibre content of the food really begins to take effect, and in people on high fibre foods, whether they're Africans or Westerners, the pellets pass quickly and easily through the colon and out into the stools. In those eating highly refined diets the pellets may stay in the colon for days and become widely separated from each other. A few may remain in the colon for a week or even longer.

These studies with inert plastic pellets help point to the potential dangers of having noxious substances in the food residues that pass through the colon. If a plastic pellet can remain in the same position against the colon wall for hours or even days, just imagine what damage a carcinogenic substance in the food residue might do in the same circumstances. As we'll see in the chapter on cancer of the colon, this is exactly what seems to happen. But for the moment let's stay with the other effects of fibre in the colon.

We've seen that fibre-rich diets mean a quick passage of waste products through the bowel; but research as long ago as the 1930s showed that in patients eating bran the volume of the stools passed was also much greater. Dr Alec Walker, working in Africa soon after the Second World War, was one of the first to be impressed by the enormous size of the stools of the people eating high-fibre diets. He pointed out that the daily weight of the stools was inversely related to the transit time. That is, people passing small, hard stools had long transit times and those passing large, bulky, soft stools had short transit times. It soon became clear that it was easy to change from one group to the other simply by altering the amount of fibre in the diet. McCance and Widdowson, the two nutritionists who conducted the barium and bread experiment, found that they could reduce the transit times of their subjects by 24 hours or more simply by asking them to eat wholemeal bread.

Despite all this evidence, experts were actually advocating low-fibre diets until the late 1960s because they thought that all forms of roughage 'irritated' the bowel and so were bad. It wasn't until about this time that some basic and crucial research was carried out by Mr Neil Painter, a London surgeon.

He looked carefully at the possibility that low-roughage diets were causing harm to the colon and might even be the direct cause of the small blow outs or 'diverticula' found in the bowels of 60 per cent of Western people over the age of 60.

Other researchers had been measuring pressures in the large bowel for about 30 years with some difficulty, mainly because their apparatus was so difficult to use and gave unreliable results. These early methods involved the placing of small balloons in the colon whose interior pressures were monitored by connecting the balloons to measuring devices outside the patient. Unfortunately they measured the pressures in the balloons which were not the same as those in the bowel. Others used open-ended, water-filled tubes which likewise were inserted via the rectum into the segment of colon being studied.

Painter's great advance, which paved the way for our modern understanding of fibre and the pressure diseases, was to combine ciné-X-rays and pressure measurements while studying the same patient. He took serial X-rays of the colon filled with barium and recorded the pressures inside the colon at the same time. This enabled him to correlate the actual anatomical and physical changes taking place in the shape of the bowel with the pressures inside it. He used this technique to see what happened when various drugs were affecting the colon and when it was stimulated by filling it with barium. These studies led to a completely new understanding of how the colon works when it is generating pressures in order to propel materials passing through it.

The colon isn't simply a five-foot-long septic tank for the body's wastes. The circular rings of muscle around the colon wall contract and form constricting rings. Two rings can close so tightly and completely that they form an isolated pocket of colon in between them. In this pocket, pressure builds up until the constricting ring of muscle at the far end opens and allows the food residue to be pumped along the bowel. This process continues along the whole length of the colon and is called 'segmentation'. It's essential for the passage of faeces along the colon – each segment contracts and relaxes in turn so the food is forced along in an earthworm type of movement.

Sometimes, the faeces are shunted backwards and forwards by changes in pressure. This happens most often in the very last part of the colon, where the faeces may be shunted back and forth several times to absorb water and make them more solid.

It was soon realized that many people on low-fibre diets had unusually narrow colons which tended to shut off very easily when producing their constricting rings of muscular contraction. This in turn produced small pockets of high pressure which gave the patients pain and discomfort and eventually made the wall of the colon blow out in several places just like an old car tyre. These small bladder-like blow outs are called 'diverticula' – hence the name diverticular disease of the colon.

Once these blow outs are formed, they never disappear and in a person on a low-fibre diet more and more appear until the colon is studded throughout its whole length, and looks as though it is surrounded by bunches of small grapes.

The reason why most of us haven't even heard of diverticular disease is because it develops quietly over many years, and can be present for a long time without causing any trouble and without the owner ever knowing. It's easily diagnosed on X-ray when the extent of the condition can be readily assessed.

Most people in the West die from something entirely different, although usually from one of the other diseases associated with eating refined foods. Hence most diverticula don't cause much trouble. Millions of others with the disease only have vague discomfort and 'indigestion', and simply take antacids or other home remedies, not realising that it's really their diverticula that are giving them trouble.

People with these narrow colons are often very constipated because their faeces are so small and viscous, like thick tar, that their colons take several days to push them through. The muscles of their colon walls have become much thicker through having to work that much harder to move their stiff contents, and their narrow-bore colons simply are not wide enough to let the faeces through easily and quickly.

But now for the great discovery. These very same people, with their pain, flatulence, bloatedness and constipation find their condition dramatically improved simply by taking bran.

More details of this later – but for now suffice it to say that bran produces much bigger, softer motions. This is because the bran fibre is dry, so that it absorbs a great deal of water. The result is that the stools are larger and softer like soft toothpaste, and pass through the colon easily without the bowel muscles having to strain. The contracting muscles in the colon wall don't have to squeeze nearly as hard to pass the stools along: pressure measurements show that the colon squeezes very gently indeed when propelling large, bulky, soft stools. The patients notice that the stools are voided more easily and they lose their symptoms because their intestines no longer have to struggle with hard, stiff motions.

So Hippocrates was certainly right all those years ago when he said 'To the human body it makes a great difference whether the bread be made of fine flour or coarse, whether of wheat with the bran or without the bran.'

Let's look more closely now at the diseases linked to 'pressure'.

Diverticular disease of the colon

Diverticular disease is the commonest disease of the colon, after constipation. To calculate how common it is, remember that the percentage of the population suffering from it is about the same as that group's age in years. This is because it gets commoner with increasing age. This rule is only true for people over 40 years old, and means that 70 per cent of 70-year-olds have the disease. When you bear in mind that there is an increasing number of elderly people in the population, you will realise that diverticular disease is a growing medical problem.

Yet as recently as 1920 diverticular disease of the colon was not mentioned in medical textbooks. This certainly wasn't because doctors didn't know what to look for, because diverticular were recognised as early as 1815, when medical opinion was that they were caused by constipation. Little did those doctors know how close they were to the truth. But generally speaking, before this century diverticular disease was reported as a 'one-off' curiosity disease. Suddenly things changed dramatically: instead of being a rare disease, diverticulitis became extremely common in the space of 20 years. A Dr Maxwell Telling of Leeds saw his first case in 1899, when none of his colleagues knew anything about it; and yet he was able to describe the disease and all its complications only nine years later so accurately that his writings are still reliable today.

Although Telling and other experts knew that the disease caused severe symptoms if the diverticula became inflamed, they thought that uninflamed diverticula did not cause symptoms; and as inflamation was so dangerous 50 years ago, doctors tried to stop infection by 'cleansing' the colon and not giving roughage to irritate the gut. In this they were wrong. Diverticular disease *does* produce symptoms. As long as the contents of the colon are soft and fluid and flow in and out of the diverticula, all is well, but if for any reason the faeces get stiffer, then problems are likely to occur.

Most of the symptoms of diverticular disease are vague and generalised, but they are at the least annoying, so that patients are only too pleased to be rid of them. The most common symptoms are nausea, a feeling of being bloated, abdominal discomfort and pain. Constipation is common and most sufferers have to strain when passing motions. A most annoying symptom is the feeling that the motion is never emptied properly. (There must be millions of people in the West suffering from such symptoms and not knowing that there is a simple cure.) But as well as producing such long-term desease, diverticula can also give rise to real medical crises that threaten life.

A blow-out may get obstructed at its neck, the point where it goes through the colon wall, and its contents become infected. This is called diverticulitis. Then the diverticulum may burst and cause peritonitis – a potentially fatal condition. This only happens in 10 per cent of patients with diverticulitis, but it is all the more hazardous to those who are old and less able to withstand surgery if their bowel perforates. This inflammation and perforation is called diverticulitis with a ruptured diverticulum.

Anything that could be done to prevent this disease itself, the symptoms that go with it and especially its dangerous complications, would be of great help to millions of sufferers throughout the West. Fibre is just such a help as we shall now see.

Medicine over the centuries has been bedevilled by fads and fancies. Certain types of treatment, both for specific diseases and illness in general, have found favour, become popular and then disappeared. Sometimes a medical fashion really is an important new discovery which catches on for a while but then becomes discredited because it can't quite live up to its early claims. More often, it's an idea which is a re-vamp of something that has been successful in the past, applied slightly differently. Fashions like these are now relatively uncommon in medicine, because with the progress of analytical research since World War Two we are able to be more critical of the real value of treatment claims.

The treatment of diverticular disease provides a nice example of this change. As it was such a new disease in the twenties, it was open to anyone to suggest what he thought might be the best cure. We've already seen that doctors thought it didn't cause symptoms, at least until a diverticulum became inflamed, giving rise to pain or a surgical emergency. Treatment was considered to be important only because it was hoped that it would prevent inflammation so that surgery, which was far from safe fifty years ago, would not be needed. Experience from operating on patients with a ruptured diverticulum showed that small particles of undigested food were often to be found near the mouth of the burst diverticulum. Seeds, bone chips and so on were so frequently found that it was assumed that these must have something to do with the cause of diverticulitis and perforation. The surgeons of the day put two and two together, made five, and suggested that it was this solid debris that obstructed the mouth of the diverticulum so causing all the trouble. This led to the recommendation of a low-roughage diet which then became the widely accepted treatment for diverticular disease for the next 50 years. Foods were strained to remove any solids and patients were fed on slops. Fruits and vegetables were made into a puree rather like modern baby foods. The results were often encouraging at first, and at least the doctors were seen to be doing something – 'resting' the colon. Unfortunately, in a disease which has its ups and downs whether treated or not, it took many years to show that this low-residue diet did no good at all. In fact it does harm, because it leads to small stiff stools that don't rest the colon but cause it to struggle and produce high pressures. In fact it is now known that this diet causes the disease!

The turning point came when Painter, intrigued by the success of bran in treating constipation, reasoned that it might also be of help in diverticular disease, especially as the two diseases go together so often. As you can imagine, for a respected London surgeon to go completely against 50 years of accumulated medical opinion, and say exactly the opposite, took some doing. It also put the onus on him to prove what he believed experimentally.

It has subsequently come to light that a handful of very well established London physicians had, in fact been using high-roughage diets for some years with good results, but they were afraid to admit it publicly in case their reputations and their practices were ruined by such unorthodox behaviour. One specialist suddenly stopped receiving patients from a colleague, although they were responding to his high-fibre treatment, because of his colleague's fear of being associated with such a revolutionary thinker: And this, at the time of the Beatles – not Bach!

But Painter was on firm ground. A close look at diverticular disease had shown him that it was rare or unknown in large areas of the world – areas where dietary fibre intake was high. Moreover, it was found that people living in these high-fibre areas developed this disease when they moved from their home country to the West, or when they reduced their fibre intake. A study of the disease in Japanese immigrants to America, and of American blacks, backs up this theory. So the differences in the occurrence of diverticular disease in various parts of the world weren't simply racial ones. Evidence pointed to an environmental change – the fall in fibre consumption.

Remember that diverticular disease was almost unknown, even in the West, until the 1920s – 40 years after the introduction of the roller mill. Until the introduction of this new machine which removed bran from flour so effectively, there was probably just enough fibre in our Western diet to keep the disease at bay. We now know that it takes about 40 years of a low fibre diet to produce the small-bore, high-pressure colon of diverticular disease. This makes it the last of the diseases to appear after the adoption of low-fibre foods.

The incidence of the disease has increased steadily in Britain during this century except during World War Two, when the death rate from diverticulitis remained static in Britain for the first time. This was when there was more fibre in our diet because wartime flour was less refined. Since then, experiments have shown that rats and rabbits fed on low-fibre diets develop diverticula, and that the pressures in the rabbits' colons were increased by eating white bread and refined foodstuffs.

As if this weren't evidence enough, it has recently been found that diverticular disease is much more common in people suffering from heart disease, than would be expected. This could be important because fibre lack may also play a part in heart disease.

Armed with all this information, it would seem foolish for doctors not to recommend high-fibre diets to patients with diverticular disease; but the pioneers in this field in the 1960s didn't have the benefit of our present knowledge. Even so, Painter went ahead with his historic study. He took 70 patients who had not improved on the traditional low-roughage treatment and put them on a diet rich in fibre. 88 per cent of them were improved and able to lead a normal life.

Painter used bran and wholemeal bread and restricted their sugar intake too. He soon found that, in spite of all the fears expressed for years, the diet didn't 'irritate' the bowel at all. On the contrary, it soothed it and improved the patients' appetites. We now know that the action of roughage in the bowel is a soothing one if anything – a fact which lead Dr Heaton of Bristol to coin the saying 'hard in – soft out'.

So effective was this treatment that the old regime was overthrown within years, and today, only six years since the first definitive article on the subject, there's hardly a physician who would dispute the effectiveness of high-fibre diets for this disease. And six years by medical standards is a short time.

Unfortunately, however good this treatment is, it doesn't do anything to cure existing diverticula. What it does though is cure the symptoms. Whether it stops new blow outs from forming is not yet known.

On a low-fibre diet the bowel seems to be able to cope with hard, viscous stools, but only up to a point. In fact the bowel wall becomes thicker and more muscular, until after 30–40 years when the blow outs begin to appear. In other words, young people's colons can handle tarry Western stools although their colons start to become abnormal from the very first days they eat low-fibre foods. The answer must be to change our diet in such a way that even a young person's colon doesn't have to strain to push food residue through. This means eating a high-fibre diet right from birth. It will also help prevent appendicitis which, unlike diverticular disease, takes its toll of children and young adults.

Appendicitis

The inflamed appendix is the commonest reason for emergency abdominal operation in the West today. The average medium-size hospital in the United Kingdom admits two cases of appendicitis every day, yet a surgeon working in Africa for five years reported that he saw no cases at all in a population of over one million people.

Appendicitis, like so many of our Western diseases, is, to all intents and purposes, a new disease. A search of all the available literature in Europe and the USA shows that between 1820 and 1840 only 33 cases were reported. Between 1840 and 1860 102 cases were seen, and between 1901 and 1918 United Kingdom appendicitis deaths doubled. A study of the medical records of the Radcliffe Infirmary, Oxford, shows that over the last 70 years the incidence of the disease has risen from between five and ten cases annually to 500 annually.

In 1920 it was remarked that doctors working in black areas of the USA almost never saw a case of appendicitis, but that soldiers, black or white, living under the same conditions had the same level of the disease. As with the other diseases we've discussed there is a direct link between the reduced dietary fibre intake and the incidence of appendicitis. Evidence for this is now so plentiful that it can no longer be considered merely a theory.

African troops in World War Two, in whom appendicitis was unknown, started to get the disease when they were issued with standard British rations. Japanese who have emigrated to Hawaii have a much higher incidence than those who stay at home, where the diet is richer in fibre.

Appendicitis seems to be the first of the intestinal diseases to appear after high-fibre eaters go on to a low-fibre diet. This has been shown most dramatically in Congolese students studying in Belgium, who had a higher incidence of appendicitis than their contemporaries studying at home. As long ago as the 1920s a famous English surgeon, Professor Rendell-Short of Bristol, noted that boys at expensive boarding schools had more appendicitis than the poorer lads at orphanages whose diets were altogether rougher. Rendell-Short also looked at Rumanian city dwellers and compared their appendicitis rate with that of their contemporaries living in rural areas and living on a largely vegetarian diet. The incidences of appendicitis were one in 221 and one in 22,000 respectively.

Dr Alec Walker, the biochemist working in South Africa already quoted, found that white prisoners suffered very much less from appendicitis than they would have done had they not gone to prison. In prison they were eating much less refined bread, less sugar and more roughage generally.

But one of the most dramatic pieces of evidence linking the disease with white refined flour comes from China, where an outbreak of appendicitis was reported in 1940 following the installation of a roller mill. The disease had not been noted in the area before, and it soon became apparent that all the cases were among government employees and students who'd got their flour from the mill. The rest of the population was still on stone-ground flour and stayed free from the disease.

Since then, studies from all over the world have proved beyond doubt that people on high-fibre foods don't get appendicitis and that those on low-fibre foods do. The curious case of the black African stevedores bears this out. These stevedores, who worked unloading ships, seemed to have a higher appendicitis rate than their families. No one could explain this until it was found that they were getting highly refined food from the ships on which they were working.

To understand how high-fibre diets actually prevent appendicitis, we need to take a look at what appendicitis actually is. The appendix is a worm-like tube the width of a pencil, and about two-and-a-half inches long. It protrudes as a little *cul de sac* from the bottom of the colon, on the right side of the abdomen.

Inflammation of the appendix can occur at any time and usually happens without warning. The hollow inside of the organ becomes blocked off for some reason, frequently by a small piece of hard faecal material, and this blockage makes the appendix swell. Along with the swelling it becomes hot and red and will eventually burst into the abdomen unless removed surgically within an hour or two. This bursting causes peritonitis which can be fatal. Because this potentially lethal little organ can burst so unexpectedly, many mountaineers, round-the-world yachtsmen and spacemen have theirs removed before they set out on their journeys, as a precaution.

Exactly what causes the original inflammation is still not perfectly understood. Over the years meat, vitamins, food processing, infection, proteins and sugar have all been blamed, but none of these can be implicated as strongly as a lack of dietary fibre. As we've seen, the faeces in high-fibre eaters are soft and flow easily along the colon. Under these circumstances, small hard pellets of faeces called faecaliths are very unlikely to form, and it is these faecaliths which are thought to block off the appendix in the first place.

A person on a low-fibre diet will have slow-moving, hard

faeces from which increasing amounts of water are absorbed and faecalith production encouraged. But we're talking about pressure diseases of the bowel and appendicitis is, after all, another pressure disease. Patients fed on wholemeal bread show an increased emptying of their appendices and those fed on low-fibre diets have raised pressures in the colon wall around the appendix. It's been known for 70 years that a raised pressure in the appendix can kill off a part of the lining. The opening from the colon to the appendix is so small, however, that any dead lining here will close it off and start infection in the 'blind' end of the appendix. Add to this the fact that low-fibre eaters have bacteria of a different kind from high-fibre eaters, and it's possible that the damaged lining might be all the more easily attacked by these bacteria.

So appendicitis, just like diverticular disease, is preventable.

Yet for all this we make a fuss about seat belts, and the link between smoking and cancer, and still ignore the lives unnecessarily lost from appendicitis. We now know the remedy – the choice is ours.

Constipation

When the average person thinks of pressures within the bowel it isn't long before he remembers the last time he strained to open his bowels. Constipation is almost universal in the Western world, but it is a particular problem in the very young, the very old and the pregnant. Constipation can, of course, be caused by serious diseases of the bowel and can even be a presenting sign of bowel cancer, so it shouldn't be ignored. Anyone with constipation alternating with diarrhoea, or constipation accompanied by bleeding, should see his doctor. Here though, we're discussing the 'normally' constipated person.

Over the centuries man has been obsessed by his bowels. When drugs were in their infancy and very little could be done to help the sick, enemas containing everything from plant extracts to port wine were widely used. For nearly two centuries the clyster or enema was a popular and universal remedy for almost all ills. People have always instinctively felt that their 'bowels' (preferably said in the same slightly guarded way as 'drains') should be opened as frequently as possible so that their bodies could be rid of the noxious 'wastes' as quickly as possible. This led to a general assumption that the normal person needs to open his bowels once a day and that we should all strive for this goal!

Because of this, the last century and a half has seen a proliferation of constipation remedies. Simple home cures, herbal remedies and other products available over the pharmacist's counter have recently been joined by the more powerful and effective products marketed by pharmaceutical companies the world over. All these remedies cost a small fortune and scarcely a home in the Western world is without at least some of them.

This would scarcely be cause for concern if all the methods and chemical substances used were completely safe – but they're not. Mineral oil, universally considered to be safe and effective, can cause Vitamin A to be poorly absorbed by the bowel. Some laxatives can cause permanent damage to the bowel wall, and the long-term use of any laxative can cause addiction to such an extent that the bowel cannot work at all without it. At this stage the bowel ceases to function in its natural way and behaves just like a drainpipe. The sufferer has unwittingly substituted laxative-induced diarrhoea for constipation, and yet considers it normal. This long-standing diarrhoea, which the laxative addict thinks an essential part of life, can be really dangerous because the passage of large-volume fluid stools deprives the body of valuable salts. If an X-ray is taken of such a bowel the irreversible damage to the colon can be clearly seen. The final price to be paid may be the removal of the colon altogether.

The treatment of these laxative addicts is difficult and time-consuming, and may need the help of an experienced psychiatrist. The unfortunate sufferer, having often been unwittingly addicted by his parents in early childhood to a daily dose of laxative, becomes obsessed with 'inner cleanliness' and ends up paying very dearly for it.

The trouble is that apart from studies on these more extreme facets of constipation, it's a subject that's been almost totally ignored by the medical profession. Most doctors consider constipation an unfortunate, but easily curable fact of life and put it down to too little exercise, the sedentary Western existence or too small a fluid intake. Most medical textbooks discuss this universal complaint as if it were of no importance, and those that do take it seriously give erroneous or misleading information. To quote from one best-selling medical textbook '. . . variations in the normal rhythm of the colon are quite wide and to evacuate the bowel twice a week is not constipation; it may be just as normal and healthy as to evacuate it twice a day'. This may well be true for populations on highly refined foods, but it is *not* the case for those eating plenty of fibre. So just as we cannot possibly accept that highly refined foods are 'natural', the bowel habits that go with them cannot be considered natural either.

So what exactly is constipation? Most people, including doctors, use the term loosely and usually incorrectly. Constipation has nothing to do with the length of time between bowel actions – it's a term used to describe the difficult passage of hard stools. True, this tends to go hand in hand with infrequent bowel action but need not necessarily do so.

After we've eaten our food all the useful parts are absorbed and the residue passed into the colon as we've already seen. If the faeces remain in the colon for long periods, they get drier as more water is absorbed by the body. They then become very difficult to pass. On top of this, any harmful chemicals either in the food residue or produced by colonic bacteria will remain in contact with the colon wall for very long periods. This can be harmful. Add to this the abdominal discomfort, tiredness and headaches that so often go with constipation, and you soon end up with an unpleasant and even potentially dangerous condition.

Having agreed then that constipation should certainly *not* be considered normal, what can be done about it? The simple answer is – eat more dietary fibre. It's almost impossible to be constipated if you're eating enough fibre . . . and enough isn't all that much. It has been interesting to see that people acting as subjects in fibre experiments have remarked, almost to a man, and quite spontaneously, that they feel so much better when their bowels are regular. This has given fibre a very good name as a laxative, and has provoked some pharmaceutical companies into marketing fibre concentrates to be used especially for patients with constipation and diverticular disease. This is almost certainly the beginning of a revolution the vanguard of which is the appearance of fibre biscuits and bran tablets, both already available. Doubtless the ingenuity of the food industry will find numerous, highly desirable ways of making us eat more bran.

So how does fibre cure and prevent constipation? Much of our knowledge on this subject comes from research done as long ago as the 1940s, when the Kellogg Company of Michigan sponsored medical research into the laxative effect of their product All-Bran. The research showed just how useful the product was as a laxative, and suggested ways in which it might act; but the medical profession was not very excited by constipation cures and the subject of roughage and constipation was dropped for some years. The public continued to eat Kellogg's bran products because they knew they worked, but it wasn't until 1942 that the subject was again looked at in a practical way by a doctor. This time it was Surgeon Captain T. L. Cleave, physician in charge of the King George V battleship, who, as we have already seen, became interested in the subject because he had hundreds of constipated seamen who could not get fresh fruit and vegatables because of the war. It was he who hit upon the idea of using unprocessed millers' bran (Kellogg's All-Bran is, as it says, all bran but it is nevertheless processed to some extent), which at that time had not been used extensively except for feeding animals. And his results were remarkable.

From 1942 until recent years dietary fibre as a means of preventing constipation was used only in a few isolated centres. Today, it's catching on like wildfire and there's no reason why constipation and other pressure diseases shouldn't be banished from the West if we were all to eat enough of it. Constipation is the first disease to disappear when fibre is added back to the diet.

Constipation is cured and prevented in three main ways by high-fibre diets. Probably the most valuable single property of fibre is its power to absorb and retain water. Food residue in the colon stays more fluid in people on high-fibre foods because of this water-binding property, which in turn makes the stools soft and easy to pass. Just put a piece of cotton wool into a jar and add some water. The cotton wool will swell until it fills a large part of the jar. Food fibre absorbs water in much the same way, and increases in bulk by as much as twenty to thirty times, which gives a much larger volume of faeces for the colon to push along. This large volume prevents diverticular disease as we've seen, and also fills the rectum with such bulk that the desire to open the bowels cannot be ignored. This in itself is important, because much of the constipation in a Western society is solely due to our ignoring the call to stool. Primitive peoples answer the call to stool at once and this helps to keep them from getting constipated. In general, it's a good principle to open your bowels as soon as nature calls.

The last action of fibre is even more dramatic. It appears that colonic bacteria act on dietary fibre to produce fatty acids. These substances have been known for years, but until recently were not thought to play a role in bowel physiology. These fatty acids, (acetic, butyric and proprionic acids) are nature's own laxatives and ensure regular evacuation of fast-moving faeces. This natural laxative effect is probably balanced by the lignin component of dietary fibre, which is thought to prevent diarrhoea. There is some evidence that fibre is helpful in diarrhoea as well as constipation but work on this is at an early stage as yet.

Almost anybody can be cured of constipation by taking more fibre in their diet, and if you're eating the sorts of foods outlined in the last section of the book, you'll never get constipated. Even the simple addition of two tablespoonsful of bran to your food every day will free you from constipation for life.

But unfortunately for those who are constipated, the twice weekly straining, pain and unpleasant sensations don't stop at the bowel. The pressures developed by the abdominal muscles in order to force the small hard stools into the outside world also produce damage elsewhere, and throw a temporary strain on the heart and circulation. Severe straining can even cause a stroke. The most common and the most unpleasant of these 'pressure diseases' is due to straining, which interferes with the circulation in the veins of the rectum, and results in haemorrhoids or piles.

Haemorrhoids (piles)

Piles are simply bulging, swollen veins within and around the anus or back passage. Half the population over fifty in the West has piles and many of them have anal bleeding, small tears and other associated painful conditions. All these can be avoided by eating high fibre foods and are indeed rare in great areas of the world where fibre is plentiful in the diet.

The chronic loss of small amounts of blood can lead to anaemia. More seriously, it may mean that a person with a cancer of the colon or rectum will put down the bleeding from these conditions to his piles, so that the diagnosis and treatment of the cancer are delayed. Any rectal bleeding *must* be treated seriously and a doctor consulted. It'll probably be something simple like piles or a small tear, but it's essential to play safe and see a doctor before embarking on self-medication. Millions of pounds are spent every year by haemorrhoid sufferers on preparations which cannot possibly cure the underlying cause. At best they can only provide temporary relief.

So what causes piles? Theories have abounded for centuries. Strenuous work, horse riding, standing for long periods, pregnancy, sitting on hot surfaces and many other things have all been blamed at various times. Unfortunately, these ideas don't hold water because there are whole areas of the world where some or all of these things are done, even done to excess, and yet piles are still rare. In most of the developing countries piles are very uncommon, yet people moving from these countries to developed ones take on this condition with their new country.

At one time it was thought that man as a species was destined to get piles because he doesn't have a system of valves in the abdominal veins that return blood to the liver (of which the haemorrhoidal veins are a part). But Africans and Asians have the same anatomy as we do and are much less troubled by this affliction – unless they eat highly refined foods. So the answer isn't a simple anatomical one.

Piles are almost certainly caused by excessive intra-abdominal pressures built up when we strain to pass our hard Western stools. The veins in the legs have valves which help the blood to return 'up hill' to the heart. The veins inside the abdomen taking blood to the liver don't have these valves, so any extremes of intra-abdominal pressure will stress them. Straining to pass a constipated motion puts a tremendous stress on the body as a whole. The pressure inside the abdominal cavity, normally very low, increases on straining to twice the normal blood pressure. Coughing can raise it to four times the blood pressure. It's no surprise then that quite a number of people suffer a stroke whilst straining to open their bowels. In response to this very high pressure, the veins in the anal area, being very thin walled and very close to the surface, simply bulge out and become haemorrhoids.

Once you've got haemorrhoids, they're there for life and need surgery or injections if they're large and give troublesome bleeding. Small piles can be prevented from progressing by adopting a high-fibre diet but no amount of fibre will cure advanced piles even though it may reduce or abolish the symptoms.

Closely related to haemorrhoids among the 'pressure diseases' are varicose veins.

Varicose veins

These swollen, twisted veins can be seen in the legs of many people. The main thing that bothers their owners is that they look unpleasant; but they can also cause swelling, pain and inflammation, and may even actually ulcerate and bleed. In short, they're a nuisance at best and potentially fatal at worst. Once more, they're rare in developing countries, but are appearing in the towns even of these countries as the rural people become urbanised. In the UK between 10 and 17 per cent of adults have varicose veins, and a study of multi-nationals in Switzerland showed an incidence of 29 per cent. Between the two of them, haemorrhoids and varicose veins cause three million lost work days a year in Britain alone.

Rather like haemorrhoids, varicose veins have been attributed to many causes. The oldest theory is probably that man hasn't yet adapted to being an upright animal, walking only on his hind legs. At first sight there seems to be some sense in this. Blood from the legs has a long way to go to get back to the heart and it's all up hill! But Nature gave us two systems to overcome this problem. Every time we walk, the muscles at the back of the leg below the knee contract and squeeze the blood up the deep veins of the thigh until most of it reaches the groin. This mechanism is called the 'soleal pump' after the big calf muscle – the soleus. The blood then flows upwards towards the heart in the long veins just beneath the skin, where it's trapped in sections by valves which allow blood to pass upwards but not downwards. So blood from the legs is pumped up into the large collecting vein in the abdomen – the inferior vena cava – from where it travels to the heart. As long as this pump doesn't fail, the one-way valves keep the blood from flowing down under gravity and all is well. Should the valves fail, the head of pressure is quite considerable and the columns of blood in the veins cause their walls to bulge and even to burst. The deforming of the vein walls renders the valves ineffective and a vicious circle sets in.

To maintain that man as an animal has failed to adapt to his upright posture in this regard, is clearly untenable, especially as millions of people, notably those in the developing countries eating unrefined diets, rarely get varicose veins yet have exactly the same anatomy as we do. It must be something else. Perhaps we in the West are of inferior stock, with a second class set of leg veins that we pass on to our children. This too is an unlikely hypothesis because the very people who never get varicose veins soon do so if they live in our society. American blacks and whites have the same incidence.

For years, long periods of standing were thought to be the cause, but this can't be true either. Prolonged standing undoubtedly makes existing varicose veins worse, but as far as we know doesn't initiate them. In fact, many rural peoples are on their feet for very long periods indeed and yet have less than one hundredth the varicose vein problem that we have in the West. Similarly with pregnancy: the numbers of babies born to women in developing countries are much higher than in the West, so if pregnancy were a cause they'd have a lot more trouble – not less.

The treatment of varicose veins to date is less than spectacular. Early cases get some benefit from elastic stockings, which simply compress the superficial veins of the leg and do the valves' job of holding back the blood. But elastic stockings aren't popular because to be of any use they have to be thick and so look unpleasant. Injecting the veins with a solution that causes a local reaction of tough fibrous tissue is a technique widely used, but doesn't produce a permanent cure. Surgery provides the only long-term cure, and it is usually combined with tying off the veins in the groin where all the leg veins congregate before entering the abdominal veins. Even surgery has its drawbacks and second operations are not uncommon.

The answer must surely lie in prevention. People on unrefined diets don't get varicose veins, so it's well worth taking a leaf from their book. On high-fibre foods, as we've seen, there's no straining to pass stools and therefore there are no surges of pressure down the leg veins. When we **strain** or cough a pressure wave can actually be felt shooting down the large veins of the legs if the valves are faulty. This is a sign widely used by doctors to test valve function.

But primitive rural people also have another protective factor – they squat when passing stools. This squatting position may help to shut off the leg veins at the groin so that no pressure can be transmitted down them. If a person with damaged vein valves squats and is asked to cough, no pressure wave can be felt in the leg veins. Our modern Western style of lavatory ensures that as we strain to pass our hard, small stools, all the pressure goes straight down the veins to damage or deform them.

For all this, damaged valves and varicose veins in themselves aren't life-threatening. A nuisance certainly, but very little real danger – unlike the clots that can form in the deep veins of the legs. Clots will form in the deep veins of the legs should the blood become more viscous for any reason

Deep vein thrombosis

This is a killer disease which can be prevented in the light of current medical knowledge. For one reason or another a small clot forms in the deep veins of the calf.

As such, this one small clot will probably give no trouble but . . . from a small beginning more clots can build up, until eventually the mass may be so long that it almost obstructs the whole vein. This may or may not be followed by an inflammation of the vein – so called thrombo-phlebitis. At any time this clot can break off, as a whole or in several pieces, and travel up the leg vein and through the heart to the lungs, where it becomes lodged in the blood vessels supplying the lungs. A clot like this in the lungs is called a pulmonary embolus, and causes the deaths of 5000 people every year in the UK alone. Evidence from developing countries shows that the incidence there is very much less than that in the West.

As there is no way of knowing if and when a piece of clot will break off and become lodged in the lungs, doctors try to prevent the clots from forming in the deep veins of the legs in the first place. These deep vein thromboses, as they're called, are common after operations (especially in the old and debilitated) and in pregnant women. This is because the blood undergoes chemical changes during and immediately after an operation (or obstetric delivery) – changes that make clot formation more likely to occur. One third of all people over forty have a deep vein thrombosis after an operation.

Many of these will never know they have had a thrombosis because they have no symptoms or signs, but the latest diagnostic techniques when used on all post-operative patients show that the clots are there just the same. Contrast this with the tiny number of Africans and Asians that get deep vein thromboses after operations in exactly the same conditions as in the West. Yet American blacks have the same incidence of clots as do their white compatroits.

Anti-coagulant drugs (like heparin), gadgets to relieve pressure on the legs during operations, leg muscle exercisers and many other methods are currently being tried so that the toll of suffering and death from deep vein thrombosis can be reduced. Yet however good the results, we can't seem to get near the low level of deep vein thrombosis experienced in the developing countries. And we probably never will, unless we eat high-fibre foods or take long-term drugs to prevent the clots forming in the first place.

Studies are under way in England to see whether high-fibre foods given pre-operatively prevent patients from getting deep vein thromboses and pulmonary embolism. Results are still being analysed but they look hopeful.

A group of doctors in Britain started putting whole wards of surgical patients on bran three times a day, four years ago. Over the four-year period there has only been one pulmonary embolus. This is a remarkably low incidence, and has led them to look more scientifically for early evidence of deep vein thrombosis using a radio-active substance that is taken up by even the smallest clot in the legs. So far, the patients on bran have been found to have much less evidence of deep vein thrombosis and none have had clinical clot formation.

So as we've seen, there's a very close link between all these pressure diseases. Haemorrhoids, varicose veins, deep vein thrombosis, constipation and diverticular disease are all linked geographically, epidemiologically and by common cause – a lack of dietary fibre.

A survey of a hundred patients with diverticular disease seen either on X-ray or at operation showed that 73 per cent of them had varicose veins. In a matched control set of patients the figure was only 33 per cent – once more pointing to a possible common factor.

Of course millions of people in the West never get any of these pressure diseases, while some unfortunate people will get them all. Is there a familial predisposition to them? Or could it be that some families are eating high-fibre diets and so protecting themselves unwittingly?

Whatever the answer, the evidence in favour of dietary fibre intake as prevention and treatment of the pressure diseases is now too impressive to be ignored.

13 Bowel cancer ... the growth of interest in fibre

Whilst the small bowel almost never gets cancers, the large bowel is the site of the second commonest cancer in the West. Only cancer of the breast in women and of the lung in men occur more often. In the USA there are more than 70,000 new cases of cancer of the colon every year, and two-thirds of these will die from the cancer.

Yet, like so many of the diseases we're discussing, this would appear to be a relatively new one, and one certainly not common before the 1920s, the time when diverticular disease of the colon also appeared. Cancer of the colon is rare in rural populations the world over, and increases in frequency as people move from villages to towns. In fact, no other form of cancer is so closely linked to urbanisation. This has been proven by studies in countries all over the world, from Africa to Finland. Some of the most interesting research shows that Japanese who move to the USA have more bowel cancer than those who stay behind in Japan, and this and similar studies of Californian immigrants prove beyond reasonable doubt that we're not dealing with a simple racial difference.

It's an amazing fact that the incidence is highest in the most heavily industrialised areas of the USA, compared with the moderately industrialised parts. Before you jump to the 'stress' theory of industrialised society, just bear in mind that Seventh Day Adventists who eat vegetarian diets have lower rates of cancer of the colon, and yet have no less stress than their American compatriots. It's even possible that people belonging to a minority religious sect may be subjected to more stress!

The more we look at cancer of the colon, just as with the other diseases we're discussing, the more the environment seems to be the incriminating factor. So let's look at the environment of the colon and see if we can get any clues.

The colon is the wide-bore, tubular part of the bowel that stretches from the end of the small intestine to the rectum. The food comes into the colon in a fluid form and gradually becomes stiffer in consistency as it passes along. The colon walls squeeze the food residue along like toothpaste in a tube, and at the same time absorb water and salts from it. The colon is essential in the control of the body's water content. Because the volume of digested juices is mostly composed of water, we would lose many pints of body fluid every day if we were to pass the fluid residue that leaves the small intestine. The colon, by absorbing water from its contents into the bloodstream, helps preserve the body's water balance.

Along with water, salts are absorbed so they too are not wasted by being lost in the stools. Bile salts, as we've seen, are reabsorbed and recirculated to the liver via the bloodstream. By the time the food residue has reached the last part of the colon it's hard and dry in Western people, and is then stored in the rectum ready for passing. In the West we don't necessarily obey the call to stool at once because it's often inconvenient, so the stools sometimes remain in the rectum and colon for very long periods. Here, they get harder still, giving rise to the condition we call constipation. But more of that later because there's one more important function of the colon we haven't yet mentioned – that of the colonic bacteria.

The human bowel has millions of harmless bacteria living inside it. They mainly reside in the colon, but are also found in the small intestine. Some of these bacteria break down bile salts in the colon and so help them recirculate into the bloodstream. Without their help we'd lose our valuable bile salts in our stools. Other bacteria synthesize Vitamin K – an essential part of our blood clotting system – while others simply colonise the bowel, so stopping noxious bacteria getting a hold. This last action is rather like that of ground cover in a shrub border stopping the weeds from taking over.

Until recently these bowel bacteria had not been very intensively studied, but today they're coming into the limelight again and fibre is the reason why.

Now we know what the colon does – let's get back to its cancer problem.

Because the environment of the colon is the food residue within it, it would seem sensible to see if there's anything in the residue in Western colons that could be responsible for all the cancers seen there. So far, we know that there are three main differences between Westernised and rural people in Africa and Asia revelant to the study of cancer of the colon. First, the urbanised person eats a lot more fat than his rural counterpart; second, his consumption of dietary fibre is very much lower; and third, his colonic bacteria are very different.

Let's start by looking at the last of these first.

A large study of the bacteria in the bowels of rural Africans, Indians and Japanese showed that they were different in type and number from those in American, British and Scottish bowels and that whilst they produce deoxycholate from bile salts (see gallstone chapter), they don't produce nearly as much. It was also found that in people on high-fat, low-fibre diets, the relative proportions of the various colonic bacteria change.

Urban man eats a lot more sugar than his rural counterpart as we've seen, but no sugar gets to the colon as it's all absorbed along with other nutrients in the small intestine.

But if sugar is not to blame nor are carcinogenic compounds in our environment, as animal experiments show. If rats are fed carcinogenic chemicals they get cancers in their colons. But, if a loop of colon is isolated so that it still has a blood supply but yet doesn't allow food through (that is a food by-pass is created) then this loop of bowel doesn't get cancerous. So obviously the cancer-producing chemicals or foods have to be in contact with the colon wall to produce their action.

It seems very unlikely that colon cancer is due to carcinogenic foods or chemicals, because if it were, we'd get cancers in our small intestines – which we don't. Cancers of the small bowel do occur, but their large bowel brothers are ten thousand times more common per square inch of bowel wall.

This points to something actually happening in the colon itself. Either it's especially sensitive to cancer-producing chemicals; or these substances don't exist until the food residue gets to the colon; or the substances are in our food but aren't actively carcinogenic until they reach the colon. Perhaps the point is that faeces stay in the colon for so long in the sluggish bowel of Westerners that there's simply more time for any carcinogenic substances to act. In practice it may well be that all of these factors play a part.

First, let's see if something as simple as the fats in our food could be the cause of our greater incidence of cancer of the bowel. It's been known for years that people on high-fibre foods tend to excrete slightly more fat in their stools. This doesn't amount to much but it's possible that the difference in fat content could be responsible for the different numbers and types of bacteria that are found in the colons of high- and low-fibre eaters. Rats bred with bacteria-free bowels don't get the cancers that normal rats get when exposed to the same carcinogens. This proves that bacteria are essential for the production of bowel tumours. It's possible that the bacteria produce a carcinogenic substance from bile salt breakdown products, but such a substance hasn't yet been isolated.

Because of this apparent link between different bowel bacteria and high fat intake some authorities feel that high fat consumption is responsible for bowel cancer. This may well turn out to be part of the story, but it's not the whole story because, as we saw in the gallbladder chapter, deoxycholate (thought to be the precursor of the mysterious carcinogen) circulates in the bloodstream and goes back to the liver and gallbladder. There's absolutely no evidence that this recirculation causes any kind of cancer either in the blood, liver or gallbladder. Perhaps deoxycholate itself is not the culprit.

One other difference in the colonic environment that could explain the cancer story is the fibre content of the food. As we've seen, there are lots of things that we still don't know about fibre, but we do know it absorbs water. People on high-fibre foods don't reabsorb nearly as much water from their colons because the fibre binds water so effectively. This means they pass larger, bulkier and softer stools and pass them more frequently. So the fibre actually 'dilutes' the stool and may therefore 'dilute' any cancer-producing substances too. Also, because the residue passes quickly through the colon, there's less time for carcinogens from whatever source to come into contact with the bowel wall. This speedy transit allows less time for the degradation of bile salts which occurs so readily when the residue is nearly static, so if there is anything in the fats and cancer theory fibre will help here too.

Recent research has shown that food residue in the colon behaves in an unexpected way. It doesn't pass uniformly along like water in a drainpipe, but certain areas 'stream' at faster rates than others. In low-fibre situations parts of the food residue can become so hard and static that they remain in one place for hours or even days. So if a hard mass did contain carcinogenic material of any kind it could well be in contact with the bowel wall for a very long time. In a person eating plenty of fibre the colonic contents flow more uniformly and backwaters of static faeces don't occur.

So combining these two arguments it seems sensible to eat a high-fibre diet and so produce rather different bacteria, a faster transit time and dilute bulky stools, together with a reduced dietary fat intake. It's unreasonable to expect people to reduce their fat intake very much, because a fat-free diet becomes al-almost unpalatable. This has been tried for coronary heart diseases which kills ten times as many people as cancer of the colon, but without success. People can't stop eating fat entirely. But then there's no reason to suppose that fat in small amounts is harmful to the colon, provided that it's accompanied by a high-fibre, unrefined diet. Increasing your fibre intake dilutes stool bile acids and so reduces the concentration of potentially carcinogenic substances.

But cancer of the colon is far from beaten. Although a high-fibre, reduced-fat diet will undoubtedly help, there's no promise that if you eat fibre you'll never get cancer of the bowel. There are probably other factors involved of which fibre and fat are just two. But until the day comes when we have the whole answer it makes sense to eat a high-fibre diet and give yourself the benefit of the doubt. After all, it can't do you any harm.

Section three
Living with your High-Fibre Diet

14 What should I eat?

Giving dietary advice is a bit like running a donkey derby . . . a problem right from the start! The trouble is that we all enjoy such different foods and have such positive likes and dislikes, and we may even have been conditioned by our past into thinking that some foods are especially 'good' or 'bad' for us. Food means so many different things to different people that it soon becomes a very emotive subject.

For years doctors, dietitians and health food faddists have been exhorting us to eat this one minute and that another. One minute the fats are all bad, the next we're all supposed to be yoghourt maniacs. So it's hardly surprising that the average man in the street is somewhat baffled. As a result, he tends to carry on in his own way, eating what he likes, hoping that by the time the experts have got themselves sorted out he'll be proven right anyway!

One of the reasons that food experts cause so much confusion is simply that they're too 'expert'. They tend to get carried away with their pet theories and forget that no one but a fanatic could possibly hope to adhere to their idea of the perfect diet. Life has to go on in spite of, rather than because of, 'good healthy foods'. Doctors find it difficult enough to get patients to take medicines properly, even when they have proven diseases for which drugs can definitely offer success. So what hope does the dietary counsellor have when the only things he can offer are doubtful and rather long-term results?

After all, there are no 'wonder' foods that can transform our lives, whatever anyone tells us. What we can do though is to try and alter our diet to that associated with a healthier way of life. This is exactly the basis of the High-Fibre Diet.

My approach to the High-Fibre Diet is based on some simple

assumptions. First, that you're not a food faddist; second, you've got a family to cope with and third, you'll want a diet that's pretty straightforward and easy to follow. Like anything new it takes a bit of getting used to but you'll soon wonder how you ever ate anything else.

There are two cardinal principles of the High-Fibre, unrefined Diet:

1 Eat carbohydrates in as unrefined a state as possible.
2 Eat foods rich in fibre whenever you can.

REMEMBER, this isn't a diet in the generally accepted sense of the word – you're simply getting back to eating what we as a species were meant to eat. Millions of people all over the world eat a diet like this and suffer few of our Western diseases, so it's obviously perfectly safe and has been well tried for millions of years. How many other diets could claim this?

The High-Fibre Diet involves eating more whole foods than you've probably done before. In general, if a food is manufactured or processed – try and avoid it.

A basic plan for healthy eating

1 Avoid white flour and its products
2 Eat as little sugar as possible
3 Eat plenty of fruit and vegetables, whole grain products, nuts and seeds.
4 Reduce the amount of fat you eat
5 Eat as few synthetic foods as possible
6 Only drink alcohol in moderation
7 Add millers' bran to your diet if necessary

1 Avoid white flour

Man has been eating grain for thousands of years. Rice, wheat, rye, barley and oats are excellent sources of the nutrients we need. Wholemeal flour is a readily available, plentiful source of protein, carbohydrate, minerals, vitamins and fibre, and it's cheap.

White flour though has been robbed of its minerals, vitamins and fibre by the process of milling and so is not nearly as nutritious as the whole grain itself. A basic principle of the High-Fibre Diet is to cut out all foods containing white flour and replace them with those containing whole grain flour.

Popular foods containing white flour are:

White breads	Biscuits
Many brown breads	Instant puddings
Rolls	Sauces
White macaroni and spaghetti	Packet soups
Breakfast cereals	Baby foods
Cake mixes	Prepared meats

Many processed foods have white flour added as a bulking or thickening agent, but unless you eat lots of them you won't be eating very much white flour from these sources.

So how can you get round eating any of these foods? Easy:

1 Don't eat them at all – they're not essential to life.
Or better still,
2 Replace them with wholemeal flour equivalents.

Because bread has always been such an important part of our daily diet, let's start with that. First, get rid of all the white flour and white bread you've got in your house. Replace them with 100 per cent stoneground wholemeal flour and bread. These are readily available in most supermarkets and health food stores.

Try making your own bread. Many people think making bread is difficult – it isn't. Follow the recipe at the end of this section, and you'll eat bread such as you've never eaten before – bread rich in nutrients and fibre and tasting wonderful. If you think it's going to take a long time to make – don't worry. It doesn't. Once you get the hang of it you'll be turning out wholemeal bread, rolls and so on like a true professional. Some people find they like to bake several loaves at one go and put the extra in the deep freeze or refrigerator. Wholemeal bread stores very well in a deep freeze and will keep for a week or more in a refrigerator. Beware of the white bread lovers who'll tell you that wholemeal bread doesn't keep. Even in a bread bin it keeps for a week. What they mean is that it doesn't have a very long shelf life like white bread with all its added chemicals. So what? Simply make smaller loaves that you *can* eat within a week.

A word about brown breads. These are usually *NOT* made of wholemeal flour. Lots of the 'health breads' would like to give the impression they are – but beware. Bread is brown for one of three reasons –

1 It's been coloured to make it look that way
2 It contains added wheatgerm
3 It contains bran

Even many of the loaves with grains stuck on top which look so 'natural' and healthy are white bread which has been coloured, and grains added for effect. You may well find that even the people selling you your bread won't know what you're talking about when you ask for wholemeal. Insist on 100 per cent wholemeal – and preferably stoneground rather than roller milled. You can have 100 per cent wholemeal flour that has been roller milled – after all it can still contain 100 per cent of the grain – but stoneground flour and bread made from it is almost certainly better because the more gentle grinding by the stones hasn't smashed up nature's grains so harshly. We simply don't know what happens to the intrinsic properties of the grains when we treat them so roughly.

So don't be fobbed off with brown loaves with added wheat germ, they don't contain the essential bran, minerals and vitamins that wholemeal breads do.

To be sure of what you're getting then, bake your own wholemeal bread, rolls and biscuits and in fact start using wholemeal flour just as you would use white flour.

What are the advantages of wholemeal bread?

1 It tastes nicer
2 It's so filling that you need less of it than white bread – so it's less fattening
3 It's rich in minerals and vitamins
4 It contains bran – rich in fibre
5 It has no added chemicals, preservatives, colourings or indeed anything else. (This is only honestly true if you bake your own – there may be a few additives to some commercial wholemeal breads, though they're not on the scale of those in white breads. Read the packet, or ask your baker before buying your first loaf, and when you find a good one stick to it.)

But lots of people eat very little bread – they've got used to eating breakfast cereals and crispbreads instead.

Most breakfast cereals are very low in fibre and are therefore mostly refined carbohydrate. To add insult to injury some even have highly refined sugar added. All these should be avoided. Cereals with bran added or those made from the whole of the wheat (look on the packet for details) are very good.

Kelloggs, the biggest name in breakfast cereals have been quick to respond to the high-fibre story and now make several high bran cereal products – some with added fruit. In fact, their product All-Bran has been available for over 40 years. These cereals are all very good and supply lots of fibre. Other manufacturers are now following suit and wholewheat breakfast cereals are to be found everywhere.

Of course you can make your own cereals. Mueslis have become very popular recently, but are expensive if bought in packet form and some already contain sugar. Look at the contents printed on the packet before buying. Make sure there's no added sugar.

Other cereals can be bought from health food stores and make tasty home made cereals, (cracked wheat, whole wheat, barley, rye or millet cereal and, of course, porridge). Porridge is rich in fibre, especially if it's one of the non-instant types.

Crispbreads first became popular as part of slimming diets. Some of them are indeed very low in calories and this is helpful if you're overweight. Here again make sure you choose one made with the whole of the wheat or rye. There are several available now and they have the advantage over wholemeal bread of being even lower in calories.

Because wholemeal bread is so filling you'll be hard pushed to get through more than four slices a day but remember that this bulk displaces other foods from your diet so you'll find it helpful in losing weight.

Today you can get wholemeal macaroni and spaghetti, which are much higher in fibre than their white brothers. Once more, they're more filling – so you need less of them.

White rice (with its bran removed) should be avoided – choose brown rice whenever possible. It takes slightly longer to cook but apart from that is better in every way.

Cakes, biscuits and puddings are luxuries, let's be honest. So if you're eating things as a luxury at least do yourself the favour of ensuring that they're not doing you any harm.

The appeal of these foods is closely linked to their sugar content – if they weren't sweet we wouldn't like them. The next section talks about sugar, but here I'll point out how easy it is to use wholemeal flour to make cakes and biscuits, and leave you to try the recipes for yourself. There are lots of delicious cakes and biscuits you can make using wholemeal flour, bran fruit and nuts. They're in no sense 'health foods' but simply taste fresh, are good for you and don't make you put on weight. If you remember that half the population is obese and then look at a neighbouring supermarket basket you'll see why. Trolleys filled high with biscuits, cakes, cake mixes and instant puddings spell obesity and unnecessary illness.

From today there could be whole areas of your supermarket that you need never see again. Don't envy the woman with the trolley piled high with refined 'goodies' – maybe she doesn't know what she's doing to her family.

The other trouble with many of the readymade, instant foods, is that in addition to white flour they contain all kinds of chemicals, preservatives and so on. We simply don't know how dangerous most of these are, so it's surely safer to avoid them if possible (see section five).

As well as avoiding white flour and all its products I should just mention the other highly refined foods which you're better off without. They're not strictly made of flour as such, but things like semolina, tapioca, sago, ground rice, arrowroot, cornflour, custard and blancmange are all best avoided *unless you add bran to them* (see section 7). As they come out of the packet they're highly refined.

2 Eat more fruit and vegetables

Along with wholemeal flour and its products, fruit and vegetables are a good source of dietary fibre. Almost all vegetables are rich in it.

Don't make the mistake of thinking that only the 'fibrous' stringy vegetables like celery and rhubarb are good. The obviously fibrous vegetables simply contain more of certain types of 'woody' fibres. Peas, beans and lentils are extremely high in fibre and yet are hardly 'fibrous' to eat.

So work on the assumption that all fruit and vegetables are good and contain fibre.

Of course they're also good because they contain other things too. For millions of people throughout the world they're the only source of sweetness. You'll be amazed how sweet carrots, sultanas, dates and even onions taste once you've stopped eating added sugar. After all, Nature intended us to eat our sugar wrapped up in fibre and when you go back to doing this you'll see how nice it is.

As vegetarians have proved over the centuries, it's quite possible to live on fruit and vegetables alone. Most of us wouldn't like it though because we've got used to eating a mixture of meat, fish and dairy products along with our fruit and vegetables. From a fibre point of view the pure vegetarian does especially well; but although he can get all the carbohydrates and proteins he'll need for a healthy life, he'll need Vitamin B_{12} to be added from somewhere or he'll get a serious anaemia. Vitamin B_{12} is only found in large quantities in meat, and especially in liver, so he'll either have to eat some meat now and again or take Vitamin B_{12} tablets every week. Even so, it's a shock to some people to learn that man can live so healthily on wheat, fruit and vegetables. Don't forget that primitive man and the higher primates were fruit and plant eaters.

Although fresh fruit and vegetables are relatively expensive, it's money very well spent – provided of course that you choose wisely and then don't ruin the food once you've bought it. We in the West seem to have perfected the art of taking nutritious fruit and vegetables and massacring them in the kitchen. More than 50 per cent of some vitamin values and 77 per cent of mineral values are lost or destroyed by excessive heating of food. Prolonged heating also probably alters the very nature of the valuable fibre vegetables contain.

Getting the most out of fruit and vegetables starts with the buying. Buy small amounts of fruit and vegetables and eat them fresh. This especially applies to leafy green vegetables which go off quickly. A few days storage reduces the Vitamin C content of their leaves by as much as 80 per cent.

Make friends with your greengrocer – he may give you bruised fruit slightly cheaper and you can use it in dishes such as fruit salad or for cooking after removing the bruised parts.

Don't buy vegetables that have been bleached, and in general choose the darker vegetables rather than the lighter.

Needless to say it's best to buy fruit and vegetables that are in season. Some freeze well, but as yet we don't know what damage this may do to the fibre content. At the moment there's no reason to believe the fibre is damaged in any way.

Always keep fruit and vegetables whole until you need them – don't even wash, slice or peel them until then.

More people are growing their own vegetables today. This is not only good fun and a rewarding hobby but it also saves money. You don't even need to have a proper vegetable garden – simply grow the odd vegetables in your flower beds in between the shrubs and flowers. Things always taste better if you've grown them yourself, and with good refrigerators and deep freezers the problem of gluts of vegetables no longer exists. Simply wrap the fruit and vegetables carefully and deep freeze them. Some freeze well and others don't – consult a good book on the subject so as to avoid ruining your home produce.

When it comes to cooking vegetables there are some simple rules:

1 Always boil water before adding the vegetables. If you put vegetables into cold water and then bring to the boil it does more harm to the nutrients than does quick boiling. Use the smallest amount of water possible, then use this for sauces, soups and stocks. Don't throw vegetable water away as it contains valuable minerals and vitamins and keeps well in the refrigerator.

2 Don't overcook. Fruit and vegetables are much nicer if slightly undercooked. 'Bubbling cauldrons' of food, especially fruit and vegetables, are not compatible with healthy cooking and must destroy the fibre to some extent.

3 Whenever possible eat fruit and vegetables raw.

4 Don't add chemicals to your cooking. If you want to keep green vegetables from going white add a few drops of lemon juice to the water. Don't use salt when cooking. Add the salt at the table if necessary. When spinach is cooked in salted water it loses nearly 50 per cent of its iron content as compared with a 19 per cent loss when cooked without salt.

5 Eat vegetables in their skins whenever possible. Wash fruit and vegetables properly first but do this quickly and without prolonged soaking. If you have to peel fruit and vegetables don't use a knife – you lose too much of the skin and often of the vegetable itself. Use a peeler that takes just the surface off. Remember – every time you peel a fruit or vegetable you're refining it and throwing away some of the valuable fibre which you've paid for.

There's little point baking wholemeal bread or buying bran if you throw away other fibre you've already bought. Potatoes should be scrubbed to remove the soil and dirt, and the eyes removed. Then cook them in their skins and eat everything. You've probably never thought of eating potato raw. Give it a try. Add some thin crispy slices to a green salad.

6 Cook so as to retain the natural flavours and aromas of the food. Steam, pressure cook, sauté or grill. Do it quickly and with the minimum of water or other additives. Don't reheat

fruit and vegetables time and again as this only compounds the felony of nutricide and further mutilates the natural fibre content.

7 Make large quantities of things like bean pot, soups or apple puree and store in a refrigerator. These all keep well and save time and fuel later when you need them.

3 Eat as little sugar as possible

Partly for historical reasons, sugar has come to be regarded as something of a luxury. Suggest to the average mother that she and her family could or should go without sugar, and she'll think you're depriving them of one of life's 'essential' luxuries. Most people realise that sugar isn't really a necessity for life, yet have become so dependent on it that they find it difficult to give up.

All carbohydrate food is converted into simple sugars by the digestive juices in the bowel, so if we're eating at all it's impossible to starve the body of the sugars it really *needs*. The myth that we need sugar for energy is a dangerous one. The only things sugar can be guaranteed to do are 1) rot your teeth and 2) make you fat. The trouble is that most animals seem to like the taste of sweet things and man is no exception. Mind you, he also likes salty savoury things, but has chosen to indulge his taste for sweet things above all the others.

Our taste for sweetness is indulged and nurtured right from infancy. This soon becomes a frank addiction to sugar and 'kicking the habit' is as difficult as stopping smoking or drinking. But just as with smokers and drinkers, once a sugar addict has cut down or stopped altogether, he feels a lot better for it.

Sugar is not a single chemical substance – there is a whole family of sugars. Nature intended us to eat sugar together with its fibre which, because of its chewiness and bulk, would mean that we'd eat very little of it. Modern sugar refining has meant that pure sucrose can now be extracted from within its protective fibre coat and used in highly concentrated forms. Ordinary table sugar be it white, brown or any other colour is sucrose, and highly refined sucrose at that. Brown sugars are no better for you than white, although it is possible that molasses might be marginally less harmful than the more highly refined sugars.

Fruits contain another sugar called fructose, and many fruits can be very sweet indeed. The most surprising things seem very sweet when you avoid adding sugar to your diet. Carrots, parsnips and onions for instance are naturally very sweet, but because your palate is overwhelmed with the high-powered sweetness of sugar you never realise they are. Most fruits are pleasantly sweet once you're off added sugar. In fact some become too sweet to take – like dates for example. Could it be that that's what Nature intended?

The trouble with eating refined sugar is that it provides enormous numbers of calories in a highly condensed form. Unfortunately, white sugar contains almost nothing else other than calories. We in the West aren't short of calories, so all the extra or 'empty' calories go to build up our body fat stores. The sugar damages our teeth if left in contact with them for long periods, and the large quantity of sugar entering the bloodstream probably damages the pancreas too as we saw in chapter four.

Sugar as such of course isn't a poison – it's a natural substance which we've refined unnaturally so that it becomes potentially harmful when taken in large amounts. We now eat over 120 lb of sugar per person per year – an enormous amount. If you find this hard to believe, just remember that manufacturers add sugar to the most unlikely foods and you'll soon see how it mounts up.

If you *can* cut out sugar altogether then do so, but if you can't, try to reduce your intake by a half or more – this will certainly help.

Here are a few tips to help wean you off sugar:

1 Start to think of sugar as a condiment and not as a food in itself. Sprinkle as little as possible on to food and soon you'll get used to the less sweet taste.
2 Try taking half the sugar you usually take in your tea or coffee. After a week of this cut down by half again and repeat the procedure until you're taking no sugar in drinks at all.

3 Reduce the amount of sugar you normally use in your cooking by half.

4 Don't add sugar to breakfast cereals – add some dates, currants or chopped fruit instead. They're sweet tasting and you'll get more fibre too.

5 Cut down on all soft drinks and beverages such as drinking chocolate.

6 Preferably get rid of all your jams, treacles and other spreads containing sugar. They only become a temptation in the early days and a nuisance later on because they take up shelf space and you never use them.

7 Stop buying cakes and biscuits. Not only are they made of refined white flour but they're usually laden with sugar too. Your own home baked biscuits and cakes (see recipes) will soon take their place. Try to think of cakes and biscuits as the luxury they always were. They were never meant to be a main source of food – which is how some people treat them today. Eat more wholemeal bread at teatime for instance and use wholemeal crispbreads or oatcakes and spread them with savoury spreads or peanut butter.

Just a word about honey. Many people imagine that because bees make honey it must be 'natural' and therefore good. Honey is made by bees and contains many different sugars. The supposedly valuable properties of honey have been acclaimed by health food enthusiasts over the centuries and they're difficult claims to disprove. However, it's only fair to say that honey is made of sugars almost entirely and so is dangerous on the tooth decay and obesity-producing fronts. True, it also contains enzymes, minerals and vitamins and it's possible that these may confer some health-giving properties, but we simply don't know for sure. What we do know is that honey, just like any other sugar, will damage teeth and cause obesity if eaten in the same amounts as refined table sugar. Its potential benefit, real or imagined, I find impossible to evaluate in the light of current scientific knowledge.

But what of the artificial sweeteners – cyclamate and saccharin? In large doses cyclamates have been found to reduce the growth rates in young animals and also to cause diarrhoea. They cause serious injury in guinea pig livers. Japanese research has proven that pregnant mice fed cyclamates have a greatly increased rate of stillbirths. So it's probably wise to avoid aboth of these artificial sweeteners and all foods containing them until we know more about them. Soft drinks and instant soft drink products (both very popular with children) are especially high in sugar substitutes, and should be avoided whenever possible because of the possible harm to growing children. Sugar in small quantities is almost certainly safer.

The best possible way to control sugar addiction is to prevent it. Start with your children and help them by example and encouragement (see chapter eight). Today's middle-aged westerner is obese and often toothless. By keeping your children's sugar consumption to a minimum you can stop them following in your footsteps – quite a thought!

4 Eat less fat

People have written whole books on this subject alone. Evidence is confused and conflicting but it seems reasonable in the light of present knowledge to reduce the amount of animal fat you eat. This means cutting the fat off meat, eating less butter and fewer fat products. In my opinion you don't need to go to the length of drinking only skimmed milk but some experts would disagree.

Eating unsaturated fats (such as many cooking oils and soft margarines) may well help reduce the levels of the blood fats thought to be of importance in heart disease.

My main reason for recommending a reduction in fat intake is that fat is our most potent source of energy. Every gramme releases nine kilocalories of energy – more than twice that in every gramme of carbohydrate we eat. Fortunately, fat is very cloying to eat and is difficult to overeat, but even so it should be taken only in moderation. Unless you reduce your fat intake a little – no matter how closely you adhere to the rest of the High-Fibre Diet – you probably won't lose weight very quickly (You'll still get all the other benefits though.)

5 Eat fewer synthetic foods

Synthetic or factory made foods are potentially harmful on three counts:

1 they are highly refined
2 they contain additives
3 they may contain sugar or artificial sweeteners

Anything 'instant' and highly processed should be regarded with suspicion. Read the labels carefully and if you don't like what you see – don't buy.

To do justice to this subject would take a whole book in itself but suffice it to say that the American National Academy of Sciences' *Chemicals Used in Food Processing* contains 300 pages of lists of chemicals present in American foods. The rest of the West is not much better.

Unfortunately, many modern western foods would not exist at all were it not for the synthetic additives. Ice cream is one such. That's why I say 'eat fewer synthetic foods'. I would be hard pushed *never* to eat synthetic foods of any kind, just as I'd find it impossible to eat a diet containing *no* fat. Both have been suggested by the 'experts' but then experts must lead very dull lives! This brings me to:

6 Drink less alcohol

The dangers of cirrhosis of the liver and the other physical and psychological deteriorations that go with alcoholism are well known. But here, let's look at alcohol in the context of the High-Fibre Diet.

Obviously it contains no fibre but does yield enormous numbers of calories. All alcoholic drinks of the beer family contain sugar. Spirits contain no actual sugar but yield large numbers of calories in the intestine.

Most of us like a drink so the choice of drink suddenly becomes important. If you're following a High-Fibre, unrefined diet, whisky is probably the best thing from the calorie point of view, taken with water. Bitter lemon, ginger ale and tonic water, like all fizzy drinks, have sugar added and so should be avoided if possible. Sweet wines and sherries contain more sugar than dry wines. Alcoholic drinks of all kinds contain 'empty' calories just like table sugar. You do get some other nutrients from alcoholic drinks, but you're also taking a large quantity of sugar.

Remember that drinks before meals may well stimulate your gastric juices and make you want to eat more than you need. This way you lose all round.

Like everything else – drink in moderation.

7 Add bran to your diet if necessary

Because we can't always control the fibre content of the food at the one or two meals a day we eat away from home, it's desirable to make up this fibre deficit by eating bran.

Bran, remember, is the outer covering of the grain and is especially rich in fibre. Wholemeal products of course have their bran still intact but refined cereal foods are devoid of it. Unprocessed millers' bran, as it's properly called, is straight from the flour mill and has not been processed in any way. It is not the same as Kellogg's All-Bran although this product is indeed a valuable and easy-to-eat source of dietary fibre.

It's so easy to add bran that you don't have to worry about not being able to get enough fibre. If you could eat whole foods and unrefined meals every day then you wouldn't need to add bran but this is the counsel of perfection and difficult to adhere to in everyday life.

Bran is a convenient concentrated form of fibre. It's available in packets from supermarkets and health stores and is cheap. Pet shops also sell it, but it's probably advisable not to buy your bran there because it hasn't been cleaned to a standard suitable for human consumption. Bran is also available as Bran Plus which also contains the wheatgerm – if you feel you'd like it.

Bran should be kept in an airtight tin in a cool part of the kitchen. It will not keep indefinitely and should be used in one to two months. Many people think of bran as being hard, dry and fibrous – and only fit for bran mash for horses. In fact it is a very light substance, chewy to eat and certainly not hard. It is not the same as wheatgerm, which is another part of the wheat grain removed in the production of white flour. Bran Plus contains bran and wheatgerm, and has therefore less bran per tablespoon than pure bran.

Although bran comes from the 'tough' outer coating of grains it's not at all hard. In fact when you first taste or even feel bran you'll be amazed how soft it feels. 'Roughage' is really a bad term and you'll have noticed that I've tried not to speak of a 'high-roughage' diet. You see, 'roughage' becomes 'smoothage' in the intestine, and fibre soothes the bowel rather than irritating it. If you want to know what bran does, then turn to chapter four (What is fibre?), and almost everything pertaining to fibre in general applies to bran.

There are lots of ways of taking bran, but first how do you know if you need it? If you're eating any refined foods you'll probably need some bran. You can use bran:

1 in your cooking
2 as bran products
3 as a 'medicine'.

Let's look at the last of these first. Bran is, of course, not a medicine. Some people though like to look upon it as if it were, and take it regularly so they don't forget. This is how you do it.

1 BEGIN BY TAKING ONE HEAPED TEASPOON OF BRAN THREE TIMES A DAY AFTER MEALS OR AFTER THE FIRST COURSE Some people find bran difficult to take dry but you can wash it down with water, milk or fruit juice, sprinkle it on your breakfast cereal, mix it in with porridge or add it to fruit, milk pudding or custard. Bran mixes well with soup, especially pea soup. Some people make up enough soup with added bran to last for several days, and then keep it in the refrigerator. If you bake your own bread, you can add one to two ounces of bran to each pound of wholemeal flour.
2 Bran may cause flatulence (wind) when first taken but this soon goes. Don't stop taking bran because you feel full of

wind – this sensation will pass in two or three weeks if you persevere.

3 After two weeks, gradually increase the amount of bran until you open your bowels once or, better still, twice a day *without straining*.

4 Remember that the amount of bran needed varies from person to person. If you eat lots of fruit and vegetables, you won't need to take so much bran. Some people find they need several teaspoonfuls a day.

FIND THE AMOUNT OF BRAN YOU NEED BY TRIAL AND ERROR . . .
ONCE YOU'VE FOUND THE AMOUNT YOU NEED – TAKE IT FOR LIFE.
BRAN IS QUITE SAFE.

Now for cooking with bran.

Bran is not very palatable to eat dry and is quite difficult to swallow, even when mixed with water. It's easier to eat though if well mixed with food, and this can be done in several ways. It has no real taste of its own and so can be added to any type of food, giving it extra 'chew' and bulk. Bran is nature's own extender, and makes food go a lot further as well as returning plenty of healthy fibre to the diet. Either add it before cooking, or mix it into the food at the table.

1 Sprinkle some on to your dry breakfast cereal and mix in well before you add milk. It goes very well with muesli, porridge or crumbled whole wheat biscuits.

2 Stir into soups, particularly thick soups such as lentil or pea, or cream soups such as chicken and mushroom.

3 Add to meat dishes, e.g. mince, hamburgers, meat loaf, rissoles and stews, either before or after cooking.

4 Stir into stuffings.

5 When baking bread you can add extra bran to the wholemeal flour, or to white flour or granary if that is all you have. This can also be done with cakes, biscuits, buns etc.

6 Add to basic crumble and pastry mixes, or mix with breadcrumbs for Apple Betty, for example.

7 Sprinkle over fruit when you put it into a pie or tart before baking, or add to stewed fruit at the table.

8 Add to milk pudding before or after cooking.
9 Add to packet cake mixes if you have to use them.

Lastly there are products which contain bran and should be eaten as frequently as possible. Wholemeal bread is obviously the major one of these foods, closely followed by bran-containing breakfast cereals.

Most breakfast cereals are not especially nutritious, but the bran-containing ones are an excellent start to your High-Fibre Diet. Manufacturers are now producing several 'whole of the grain' cereals – look at the packet, it'll tell you. Clearly the 'whole of the grain' means the bran too. Other more obviously bran-containing breakfast foods are also good. Some have raisins added, which means that the natural sweetness of the fruit makes it less likely you'll want sugar.

Some people put bran on top of their breakfast cereals – even if they contain added bran already!

Practical note: When eating bran, or indeed a high-fibre diet generally, it's probably wise to step up the amount of fluid you drink. Dry forms of fibre like bran and wholemeal bread absorb enormous amounts of water and this has to come from somewhere. If a reasonably high-fibre diet doesn't seem to be giving the right number of bowel actions a day – take more fluid and see if that helps.

So you can see there are lots of ways of using bran in your everyday eating. It's also useful to take away with you when you go on holiday, into hospital or to any other place where you have to lose your High-Fibre Diet for a while.

But for all this, some people either don't like, or simply can't get on with bran. Today there is no reason to miss out on such an ideal concentrated source of fibre because the food and drug companies are coming up with products for just these people.

Bran tablets are easier to take away on holiday, for example, than bags of bran, and there are concentrated fibre drinks available through doctors. These are used mainly for treating medical conditions, but can also be used on the odd occasions when you can't eat your normal High-Fibre Diet.

In an ideal world we shouldn't have to add bran to our foods, it should never have been removed in the first place. But in practice there's little likelihood of changing the eating habits of the western world overnight, so the answer must be to choose foods as rich as possible in fibre and then add any more that's necessary in the form of bran.

15 High-Fibre Diets and slimming

Food refining concentrates carbohydrates, so that more calories are contained in a given volume of food. Many of us are addicted to refined white sugar and this will inevitably lead to obesity over the years.

High-fibre foods tend to encourage weight loss because:

1 As you eat them the chewing needed produces large amounts of saliva which distends the stomach. Once the food is in the stomach further digestive juices are added and the fibre swells, so giving a feeling of fullness. Most people on slimming diets never feel full, so this is a real plus.

2 They are actually more difficult to eat. They take a lot of chewing and very often this and the feeling of fullness they produce mean that the slimmer stops eating long before he otherwise would have done on refined foods. High-fibre foods are more satisfying to chew and eat.

3 They are so bulky. Just bear in mind that you have to munch your way through four large apples to get the same number of calories as from a small chocolate bar, and you'll see what I mean. Sugar and carbohydrate wrapped up in nature's fibre take a lot of eating – just as they were meant to.

4 There's evidence that fibre actually prevents small amounts of energy from being absorbed from the intestine, and that

5 people eating them excrete more fat in their stools than do those on a low-fibre diet. As fat is our richest source of energy per unit of food, this must be a help too when it comes to weight loss.

Recently, a study has shown that eating more than a pound of potatoes every day, in addition to whatever other food they could manage, caused a group of people to lose weight over a three-month period. The potatoes (and the same is true of wholemeal bread) so satiate the appetite that there's very little room left for anything else.

If you're going to try the potato or wholemeal bread diet remember that the potatoes must be cooked and eaten with their skins and that you must not lavish the bread with thick butter or indeed any jam. The principle is that you must eat the 1 lb of potatoes or ½ lb wholemeal bread every day in addition to whatever else you can manage. This isn't of course as good as cutting down on all refined foods, but could be a good way of starting your slimming programme.

The greatest advantage of a high-fibre diet in slimming are:

1 It's perfectly natural – you don't eat large amounts of boring foods (yoghourt, skimmed milk, grapefruits or whatever) so often called for by other diets. All you're doing is changing your diet back to what it should have been all along.
2 You're never constipated – a common side effect of many diets.
3 Provided you combine it with a small reduction in fat intake, you'll get results within a few weeks
4 It's not a 'five-minute wonder' diet. Once you're on it, you're on it for life and will soon stabilise to a suitable body weight for you. It's not a fad – more a way of life.
5 It's easy and enjoyable. It's not a prohibitive diet – the only difficult part is giving up sugar. It's probably fair to say that in the light of very recent research you'll lose weight if you cut down your sugar intake by as little as a half. So even the loss of sugar shouldn't be too hard to bear.

The high-fibre diet is very much a 'Thou shalt' and not a 'Thou shalt not' diet.

Ten things to expect from your high-fibre unrefined diet

1 Flatulence (wind) and fullness. Don't be put off, this goes within two or three weeks.

2 Regular bowels with no straining.

3 A slow loss of weight.

4 Greatly reduced levels of tooth decay and gum disease.

5 A small fall in blood cholesterol level (may help prevent heart disease).

6 Increased excretion of fat in the stools (helps lose energy from the body).

7 Decreased likelihood of becoming diabetic, especially in middle age.

8 Less painful piles if they are already present.

9 Reduced colon pressures, so reducing the likelihood of diverticular disease.

10 Altered cholesterol metabolism which favours NO gallstone formation.

16 High-Fibre Diets in everyday life

Feeding your children

There's no doubt that starting a high-fibre diet in adult life *will* be beneficial, but nothing like as valuable as starting right from birth. A child that has never been used to sugar and highly refined foods has a head start over the rest of us.

So your children should be your main concern, and there's plenty you can do to start them off on the right track from day one. Unfortunately the very first drink a child has is often glucose water in the Obstetric Unit. Unless the baby is ill or premature, plain milk or water is just as good and will not start off his sweet tooth.

Baby foods

1 Breast milk is *the* best food for babies. Try if you possibly can to breast feed your baby, and do not be put off by friends and relations who may be discouraging. It is hygienic, on the spot, always available, and best for your baby and you. It is now thought that several diseases are substantially less common among breast fed babies compared with those that are bottle fed.

2 Keep sugar out of the child's diet for as long as you can. When he starts to have a mixed diet, give him what you and the rest of the family eat, put through a sieve or mouli. Vegetable soups, vegetables of any kind mixed with gravy, stock or water, and stewed fruit all go down well.

Later on you can add some meat which can also be put through the mouli or liquidised. When you choose commercial baby foods, try to select ones without added cereal or sugar because both of these will be refined. Unfortunately they are few and far between. Making your own baby foods is not only healthier but probably cheaper too.

3 Give wholewheat cereals if possible, without extra sugar, and try not to start cereals anyway until four or five months at the earliest. For older babies, instead of bought rusks make your own from baked fingers of wholemeal bread. Babies love these and the wet droppings don't stick to things like commercial rusks.

4 Fresh fruit is usually popular, particularly mashed bananas, and there is certainly no need to add sugar to these, though many people do. Cook stewed fruit with as little sugar as possible. If you must sweeten with something, add honey which goes further and may be healthier than table sugar. Remember you're not feeding yourself so you don't have to please your palate. You've become addicted to sweetness – give your baby a chance *not* to.

5 Just give your young baby milk to drink. If he is especially thirsty give him water between feeds. Keep off commercially sweetened drinks which are full of sugar or cyclamates, and are often not really thirst quenching anyway.

The baby who is being bottle or breast fed will need vitamin supplements. Fresh orange juice provides vitamin C, but some mothers find it fiddly and expensive. Most people use concentrated orange juice and cod liver oil, or Children's Vitamin Drops. The concentrated orange juice should be given in dilute form as a straight drink from a bottle or a spoon. Sweetened drinks put into a dummy and left in the baby's mouth for a long time cause dental decay and should not be used.

Children's food

People tend to equate sweet things with love and affection, and TV commercials encourage this. A mother who is strict about sweets and cakes is thought by many to be depriving her child of love. In fact the opposite is the truth. The modern habit of giving children sweets, lollies and cakes is often the result of commercial brainwashing and also a way to obtain a quiet life. I am not denying that children like sweets given the chance, but we all know that sugar causes tooth decay, makes people fat, and may cause other problems in the long term.

If you want to give your children treats, buy fruit instead. Cherries, pineapple, peaches and pears are popular with children. A fruit flan with candles round it can make a novel and delicious birthday cake.

Be strict about sweet eating – if they are going to have them let them have them after a meal, or even better still only once a day. Ideally, children (and adults for that matter) should clean their teeth after every meal. This will help prevent tooth decay.

It needs some perseverance on the parents' part to wean children off sugar, but it can be done, and most of us have only to open our mouths to show them our fillings as a reminder of *our* sweet-eating days. We all dislike visits to the dentist, and once we have fillings we have to keep going back just to repair the ones we already have.

Make a visit to the greengrocer a special expedition for a treat, instead of going to the sweet or cake shop. Let children choose a fruit or vegetable for tea. They enjoy colourful plates of vegetables like carrots, tomatoes and cucumber, and they're all ideal finger foods. Make baking into an enjoyable session so that the children have fun and will be eager to eat the end product.

Cakes were traditionally made only for special occasions, not for tea every day, or even every weekend. Why not go back to this custom, and for tea time have wholemeal bread and butter as a rule or wholemeal crispbread if the children want biscuits. Wholemeal biscuits are the least sweet of all biscuits.

Sometimes the only way is to be ruthless and to run out of things like squash, biscuits and white bread, and only have wholemeal bread in the house.

Sweets, lollies and sweet drinks eaten between meals cause dental decay, take away a child's appetite for the better foods eaten at main meals, and can also be eaten so easily that a lot of extra calories are taken in, so causing obesity in many children. Don't be afraid to be strict about them – children are reasonable if you explain your thinking clearly. Although they'll moan at you in the short term, they'll be very proud of their teeth and slim figures later on.

It's often not easy though. Children don't live only at home, where you can have complete control over what they eat. When they go to school they'll meet other children whose parents don't forbid sweets or eat whole, unrefined foods. This presents real difficulties because you as the parent can all too easily become an ogre in the eyes of your children and their friends. This takes careful handling. The watchword is *moderation*. Don't be too dogmatic – sugar isn't a poison and the odd piece of white bread won't harm anybody. Bear in mind that forbidden fruit always tastes best and you can't go far wrong.

School snacks

Children who set off for school after an early breakfast are often very hungry by mid-morning and looking for a snack. Nuts and raisins are a popular satisfying snack, also peanuts plain or roasted, dried fruit such as apricots and of course fresh fruits, carrot sticks and wholemeal crispbread biscuits. These last can be eaten plain, or buttered with a thin Marmite or cheese filling.

Many children like to take sandwiches for lunch and these can form a very nourishing and satisfying meal. Use wholemeal bread and try to include some protein filling in some of them, such as egg, cheese or meat. Give them something to crunch like raw carrot or celery. A piece of fruit is a good end to the meal.

Tea-time foods

Children home from school are often starving. Wholemeal bread and butter, toast, sandwiches, bread and banana, scones, date and walnut loaf are always popular.

Children's party foods

If you have the time, make the party food at home with wholemeal flour – if not, buy wholemeal bread and make interesting sandwiches and buy savoury foods rather than sweet ones.

A few ideas: (*also see recipes*)

Sandwiches with wholemeal bread and savoury or sweet fillings, Marmite whirls, sausage rolls and cheese straws are great favourites. Today's child seems to be very keen on savoury snacks – latch on to this while you can. Sandwiches – date, date and walnut, apple and walnut, cheese, cheese and apple, lettuce, tomato, cucumber and cream cheese, cheese and ham, cream cheese and chives, and banana all go down well.

Biscuits, cakes, pastries, rock cakes, and fruit slices can all be made with wholemeal flour.

A fruit cake can be decorated with nuts in the initial of the child, or with his age in years. These can be put on before baking. Leave off the icing and decorate (if you must) with marzipan only. Fruit flans decorated with candles and cream make an original birthday 'cake' too. If you make jelly, add lots of fruit to it.

I don't think sweet foods should be completely forbidden. They are the sort of thing that should be kept for treats and parties – we all enjoy treats on birthdays and special days. It's the everyday consumption of refined carbohydrate fun foods which needs to be drastically cut down, particularly in the diet of growing children and adolescents.

Entertaining

Once you've been converted to high-fibre, unrefined foods you'll be very loathe to go back to your old ways. Things like white bread and sweet sugary foods may well become even positively unpleasant to you.

Unfortunately not all your friends and relatives will share your views – mainly because they simply don't know about high-fibre foods and haven't tried them. This produces something of a dilemma. Should you force your strongly held views on to friends and relatives or should you go back to your old style cooking when you have guests?

My answer is that guests provide a wonderful way of

spreading the healthy eating habit. The secret though is to do it very gently and subtly.

1 Never be dogmatic – after all it's a free world and people don't have to agree with you.
2 Take trouble to plan the meal ahead carefully so that it's well balanced and not in any way 'health faddy'.
3 Choose your favourite recipes – they're probably the things you do best.
4 Don't talk about people who eat sugar and other refined foods as though they were lepers.
5 Teach by example. A really delicious meal sells itself.

The beauty of so much of the High-Fibre Diet is that it's so simple. It's also very filling so when entertaining you need less of everything. A slice of wholemeal pizza fills a very big gap and is cheap to make.

Fruit can be served raw and so saves time in preparation. What a novelty to have really nice fruits instead of a pudding. Take trouble to choose the fruits carefully and perhaps get unusual ones. Although fruit is relatively expensive it's certainly no more so than a special sweet dish for a dinner party.

If you have people in for tea or coffee, beware. These are the times when highly refined buns, sugar rolls and sweet pancakes come into their own. Buy wholemeal biscuits and cakes if possible or bake your own – it's so simple (see recipes). If you haven't time to cook from scratch, use packet cake mixes and add bran before baking. This isn't as good as using wholemeal flour but is quite good in emergencies. Two heaped tablespoons of bran mix easily into a packet mix for scones or cakes and help towards replacing some of the fibre. Lighter cakes such as sponges don't seem to fare so well with added bran.

When you have people to stay I think they ought to accept what you are eating as a family – and it doesn't take long for them to realise that eating wholefoods means simpler eating, with more colour, texture and satisfaction. Often when children come to tea they say – 'Oh, I never eat brown bread' – and before the meal is finished they have usually had two or three slices of wholemeal and really enjoyed it.

There is no need to have lots of cakes and biscuits – if people are hungry they will eat what is available, and if it is only bread, that's fine. Refined foods such as biscuits are always tempting and one goes on eating them greedily and un- necessarily, taking in far too many calories and putting on inches.

So whether you're eating high-fibre foods or not, remember that guests in your home don't necessarily want to be sold a new way of eating. Let your cooking speak for itself.

Eating away from home

Whether you're at someone's home or in a restaurant, try to keep to the sorts of food you usually eat on your High-Fibre Diet. At friends' you'll obviously have to eat what they do, but this is unlikely to be any hardship. The only thing that can be really unpleasant is having to eat sweet things when you've become used to not eating added sugar. Politely accept small portions of these foods if you find them too sickly but otherwise eat what everyone else is eating. If you happen to be a vege- tarian it's probably kind to warn your hostess a day or two before the dinner so she can make other arrangements for you.

But most of us eat out in canteens, restaurants or cafes almost every day. This is a much more serious business, because if you're eating more than one meal a day away from home it can be very difficult to keep up with your High-Fibre Diet.

Always try and choose foods high in fibre that are not too processed or refined when eating out, especially if it's every day at a works canteen or restaurant. Obviously it's going to mean that your fibre intake will fall, but you can overcome this by adding extra bran to your breakfast cereals or even by taking bran to work with you to sprinkle on your food.

Obviously if you're taking sandwiches for lunch, they'll be in wholemeal bread so you'll have control over that; but for most of us who have to eat out we simply have to accept it and take extra bran or fibre foods at other times of the day. Because many people feel they want something to fill this fibre gap and something that they could take away on holiday with them, a

British company is manufacturing fibre tablets. Once you've been on a High-Fibre Diet for some time you'll find that even a day or two off it will make you constipated. For this reason its probably best to take some bran with you if you're going to be away more than a few days.

I think it's important to stress to friends that the family is not completely obsessional about *never* eating white bread or cakes or puddings, because obviously there will be times when you go out or away to stay when you will have to eat them. If you make a great thing about it you will never be asked anywhere. People tend to have a very strong reaction when you start showing any particular interest in food, and immediately label you as a 'health food' crank, or say that you are a 'food faddist'. The way to reply is that you are neither, but think that it is important to eat 'wholefoods', ones that have not been processed and messed about by manufacturers. In some towns the only place you can buy wholemeal flour is the health food store – which is unfortunate, because they do sell a lot of foods that could be called 'cranky'.

A word of caution. Don't become a food bore! People who aren't interested in food as a way to better health can't be expected to be enthusiastic about your High-Fibre Diet. I hope that like me you'll be so convinced of its value that you'll want to 'convert' others to something you enjoy. But do be careful not to overdo it. More people have been put off valuable dietary advice by over-enthusiastic zealots than are turned on to it.

The proof of the pudding is in the eating – let people try for themselves.

Convenience foods

The whole-food cook must learn to 'think fresh' and to get away from simply opening packets and tins. Of course, there are times when you can't get to the shops or have unexpected visitors, and this is when convenience foods are so useful.

What exactly are convenience foods? They're mainly foods presented in such a way as to save time shopping, preparing and cooking. The whole-food cook can certainly make use of some of the convenience foods available, but she has to be selective, and critical in what she buys. As you get into the way of cooking with high-fibre foods you'll find your shopping basket at the supermarket is lighter, but the one at the green-grocer heavier.

Here are a few ideas.

1 Cereals

These are widely used at breakfast time and provide a quick breakfast for the family. When buying cereals look for ones which contain the whole of the wheat, or ones with extra bran added. There are one or two which contain no sugar at all, such as puffed wheat, but most others have had some sugar added in the preparation. Sugar-coated ones should be left on the super-market shelf, and there's really no need to add extra sugar to your plateful of cereal on the table. Start by putting on half the amount you usually use, and gradually reduce it week by week. Soon you should be able to eat your cereal without any sugar, and find it just as delicious.

Bran flakes or wholewheat flakes make a delicious crunchy topping for stewed fruits, and can also be used to make a flan case.

Porridge Oats can be used as a binder instead of breadcrumbs when making hamburgers, stuffing and also for toppings for fruit puddings; and oatmeal is another useful thing to have in the cupboard.

2 Canned foods

These are a great standby and keep for a long time in the store cupboard. Be selective in the ones you buy – avoid concocted meals in tins, these usually contain all kinds of extras, most of which are refined. If you must use them, add them to freshly cooked vegetables, which have more fibre and flavour. You can always add bran of course.

Canned vegetables: Tinned tomatoes are the most useful vegetable to have in a stock cupboard. Use them for soups;

add to mince for spaghetti sauce, and for pizza topping. Tomato puree in tubes and tins is also useful for flavouring. Use sweet corn for fritters and butter beans or green beans for a hot vegetable or salad. Beetroot, baked beans and spinach are useful to have in tins. In fact most tinned vegetables are good. But bear in mind that many are not as rich in fibre as their fresh brothers. Special kinds of vegetable strains are bred for their ease of peeling and canning, and some of these are lower in fibre than their 'old-fashioned' relatives.

Canned fruit: Most fruit in cans is in heavy syrup, although a few varieties are beginning to appear in natural juice and these are the ones to look out for. If you do buy fruit in syrup, pour off the syrup before use, and make fresh juice by squeezing an orange.

Canned Fish: This is useful for salads, kedgeree, fish cakes, etc.

Canned Meats: Have a look at the label. You'll find most canned meats contain a long list of extras including cereal binder, so choose the tin which is the most meaty. The same applies to savoury paste, spreads and patés – start looking at the labels a bit more – you'll be surprised what you find!

3 Stock cubes

Meat and vegetable extracts all come in useful for making home-made soups and sauces, also for cooking rice and vegetables, and for casseroles.

4 Freezers

A freezer is really useful for the wholefood cook, but of course not everyone has one. Even a small one can contain some frozen vegetables, however; and if you bake your own bread that too will keep very well for months in the freezer. Pastry for flans, quiches and pancakes can be made when you have a baking session and then stored in the freezer.

As more people are growing their own vegetables the extra vegetables can be frozen for later use. This is especially useful because crops tend to come all at once, particularly in August and September.

Frozen foods are one of the most useful convenience foods. Frozen fruit, vegetables and fish are all useful and are all whole foods. However, more and more ready-made dishes which have been frozen are filling the freezer shelves, and these contain a mass of extra ingredients, so avoid them.

5 Dried fruit and vegetables

Onion flakes, peppers, peas, beans etc. are all useful.

Dried-fruits – these are useful in store cupboards and can quickly be incorporated into cakes and puddings, e.g. mixed dried fruit, prunes, apricots, dates, etc.

6 Packets

I would suggest that you use these only in real emergencies. There seem to be more and more packets on the shelves – puddings, cakes, breads, ready-made meals to which you just add water or milk. There is no doubt that a cake out of a packet is very easy and quick to make, in emergency, and it can be given more substance by adding bran when mixing. Bran mixes well with pastries and scones, but not so well with a light sponge mix.

Boil-in-the-bag rice is convenient, but once you have eaten brown rice you will find instant rice a poor substitute. Bran mixes well with boiled rice or rissoto.

7 Drinks

Fizzy drinks, squash, syrups, fruit juices and malted drinks are all high in sugar content and are some of the easiest ways to consume unnecessary calories. They are not usually very thirst-quenching either – the best thirst quencher is water. Bring your children up to expect water to drink and to expect squash only on very special occasions.

Shopping

Plan your shopping list before you go out.

1 Make an approximate menu list for the next few days, and a list of ingredients you need to buy as you go along. A little

forward planning will mean you'll use fewer of the expensive and highly refined convenience foods.

2 Try to shop for several days at a time, if not for a whole week. Use your refrigerator or deep freeze to the full. There's no point in having these expensive machines sitting around half empty, eating electricity.

3 Try to shop by yourself. You are the person who has planned the meals for the family and you know what you want to buy. A crying child at your elbow will often persuade you to buy something for peace and quiet, particularly at the sweet counter at the end of it all.

4 Be strong-minded and walk quickly past the 'treat foods' which so many people regard as daily necessities these days – e.g. fruit squashes and fizzy drinks, biscuits, chocolates, puddings, cakes and buns and sweetened dairy products. After a while you'll simply pass them by without a second thought.

5 Costwise it probably balances out in the end, because you will gradually eat a simpler diet, and what you do *not* spend on cakes, biscuits and fizzy drinks goes on more fresh foods and the slightly more expensive wholewheat flour, pasta, rice, etc. Shop around for the wholewheat products. The prices vary from shop to shop and are usually cheaper in the supermarkets or in shops which are not also selling 'health foods'.

6 Buy flour in bulk if you are going to bake your own bread – it's much cheaper. Muesli base is also cheaper in large packets.

When you bake bread, make as many loaves as you can at a time and wrap them in foil and keep in a cool place, in the fridge, or freeze them if you have a freezer. Similarly, when baking pastry make extra flan cases and store in a tin or freeze. This saves on the gas or electricity bills. Even your own 'production line' should have economic advantages!

7 Make friends with your greengrocer – you may then get bruised fruit slightly cheaper and this can be put into fruit salad. Buy fruits and vegetables when they are in season and therefore a bit cheaper. Grow some of your own vegetables – in a vegetable plot or dotted around in the flower beds.

8 Get used to reading packaging. Look for the words 'wholemeal', 'whole of the grain' or 'wholewheat'. Try to

avoid foods with artificial flavouring and colourings, and beware of foods which contain cereal as a binder as this will be white refined flour. Lots of foods contain added sugar – try to avoid them.

9 *Don't* feel that you need to shop in health food shops. This is not necessary. You can get all the good foods you need in ordinary shops.

10 When you get to the checkout – give your trolly a final look over. Ask yourself 'Have I got any refined foods here that I shouldn't have?' Be strong willed – take them back. After a few times you won't even pick them off the shelf.

11 *Remember* you are the boss. Manufacturers will make and sell what you demand. Keep up the pressure on your supermarket manager – if enough people ask for something he'll stock it.

Your stock cupboard

Should have	*Should not have*
	(If you especially like a few of these foods – provided they do not contain sugar – eat them with added bran)
Wholemeal bread and/or rolls	White bread, rolls, pastries etc. 'Slimming' breads.
Wholewheat pasta spaghetti macaroni lasagne (green)	White pasta spaghetti macaroni etc.
Whole (brown) rice – long Whole (brown) rice – short	White rice, boil-in-a-bag rice
100% Wholewheat flour	White flour (keep a small packet of plain white flour for sauce if you must)
Oatmeal Porridge oats	Instant breakfast cereals

Wholewheat crispbreads	Most cheese biscuits
Digestive biscuits	Sweet biscuits generally
Wholewheat cereals (see	Sugar-coated cereals
packet) e.g. wheat	Cereals which do not say 'whole'
flakes, All-Bran (or	on the packet or that do not say
other bran-containing	that they contain bran.
cereals)	
Muesli (homemade)	
Salt	
Sugar – all sugar is the	
same, be it brown, white	
etc. You do need to use	
some sugar, sometimes	
honey – useful for fruit.	
A little goes a long way.	
Jams – homemade if	Jelly-type jams and marmalades
possible. If not, choose	
those made from fruit	
with skins, e.g.	
blackcurrant, coarse-cut	
marmalade.	
Tinned fish	Readymade meals in tins
Tinned meat	Most tinned meats
Tinned pastes and paté	
Tinned fruit in natural	Fruit in heavy syrup
juice	Tinned puddings, in general
	packet puddings
	Semolina, tapioca, custard powder
	sago, blancmange, ground rice
	Sweet sauces and toppings
Herbs and spices	
Tinned vegetables, e.g.	Instant potato, creamed
tomatoes, beans, corn	vegetables or vegetables in sauce
spinach	
Nuts, dried fruit (dates,	Crystallised fruits
figs, currants, prunes)	
Frozen fruit	Readymade meals in
Frozen vegetables	tins, packets or frozen

Frozen meat	
Frozen fish	
Fresh meat	
Fresh fish	
Dried pulses, peas, beans, lentils	
Tinned and frozen fruit juices (natural, unsweetened)	Fizzy drinks squashes
Fresh fruit and vegetables	Any form of 'instant' vegetables
Eggs	
Cheese	Processed cheeses
Milk	Tinned milk, sweetened yoghourt condensed milk
Unsweetened chutneys and unsweetened pickles	Sweet chutneys, sweet pickles, mincemeat
Clear soups, home-made soups	Packet soups. Tinned soups are better, since they may contain a little fibre. Bran can be added very easily.
Butter, margarine, cooking oil (other vegetable oils)	

What will it cost?

About the same – in short. Although wholemeal foods cost slightly more than the mass-produced, refined equivalents, you need less of them to make you feel full. One good slice of wholemeal bread for instance will make you feel as full as two or three slices of white bread.

As you walk around the supermarket you'll be passing by all the expensive, lavishly packaged ready-to-eat meals, cakes, pies, pastries and frozen desserts. What you save here you'll spend at the greengrocer.

Assuming that you and your family eat few or no sweets – that'll save a lot of money too.

Alcohol is expensive and you'll be downing less of that too, so there's bound to be a saving here.

You'll be eating less fat, so here again there's a saving. Cream is expensive. You'll be amazed how soon you'll go off cream once you reduce your fat intake even a little. And after all, the sort of puddings you'll be eating won't be crying out for cream. You can't drink it by the glassful so you'll probably end up eating very little at all.

Salad vegetables and crispy things to peck at when you feel hungry between meals aren't expensive. If you take up growing your own vegetables and fruit, or even buying in large amounts during the season and freezing them, you'll save money too.

Fresh fruit can be pricey, but if you shop wisely it needn't be too bad.

By and large it's fair to say that specialist stores and health food shops are more expensive than the big supermarket chains. Whenever possible buy from big stores which can pass on the benefit of their bulk buying to you the customer. There's absolutely no need to pay more for healthy food.

Beware of health food gimmicks – look twice to see what you're paying for. There's nothing magic about healthy eating and it certainly shouldn't cost a lot.

17 Some delicious high-fibre recipes

Index to recipes

Soups 196
Meat stock
Croutons for garnishing
Tomato
Split pea
Mixed vegetable

Lentil
Onion
French Onion
Mushroom
Leek and potato

Meat 199
Hamburgers
Meat loaf
Moussaka
Stuffed shoulder of
lamb
Macaroni cheese with
vegetables

Stew and dumplings
Fish with rice
Vegetables with rice
Stuffed marrow
Stuffed peppers
Stuffed tomatoes
Stuffed cabbage leaves

Vegetables 205
Potatoes – boiled
Potatoes – roast
Potatoes – dauphinoise

Potatoes – casserole
Pan hagerty
Cabbage casserole

Salads 207
Cabbage
Rice
Chicken and chicory
Cheese and apple
Tuna
Simple cabbage

Beetroot and bean
Tomato rice
Potato
Other simple salads
Cold stuffed tomatoes

Beans and lentils 212
Haricot mutton
Butter beans in sauce
Bean pot
Haricot beans with onion
and tomatoes
Lentils
Lentils and bacon

Pizza, pancakes and fritters 215
Pizza dough
Pizza sauce
Suggested toppings for
pizza
Pancake batter
Suggested fillings for
pancakes: savoury
Suggested fillings for
pancakes: sweet
Yorkshire pudding
Corn fritters
Vegetable fritters
Fruit fritters

Oatmeal 218
Herrings or mackerel in
oatmeal
Oatcakes
Oatmeal stuffing 1
Oatmeal stuffing 2
Porridge

Puddings with fruit 220
Stewed fruit
Fresh fruit puddings
Yoghourt and fruit
Crisp flan case
Crispy blackcurrant
flan
Crispy gooseberry flan
Fruit crumble
Crunchy oat topping for
stewed fruit
Gooseberry crunch
Apple Betty
Baked apples
Blackberry and apple
dumpling
Apple flan
Basic apple puree
Apricot and apple flan
Blackcurrant flan
Strawberry flan
Mincemeat and apple
flan
Fruit tart
Fruit slices
Apple balls

Rice pudding 227

Pastry 227
Basic pastry recipe
Pastry flan cases
Suggestions for savoury
fillings for flan cases
Sausage rolls
Sausage pie
Marmite whirls
Cheese straws

Tea-time foods 230

Apple cake
Tea cakes
Date and walnut loaf
Banana bread
Brown scones

Rockcakes
Nut cookies
Fruit cake
Oat cookies

Bread 235

Wholemeal bread

Wholemeal rolls

Muesli 236

Uncooked muesli 1
Uncooked muesli 2

Cooked muesli 1
Cooked muesli 2

Recipes by Dr Susan Heaton

This selection of recipes includes many of my favourites which have been collected over the past few years. The quantities given are usually enough for four people unless otherwise indicated. I have included a number of recipes using wholemeal flour for tea-time foods, pastry, pizza, pancakes and bread. These will help you to get started on baking with wholemeal flour, and then you can adapt your own recipes to use this flour and a lot less sugar. I haven't included many meat dishes because these don't usually contain refined foods; but I have given two recipes for oatmeal stuffing which is good with roast chicken, stuffed shoulder of lamb and beef olives.

When you are cooking always try to use as many fresh vegetables and seasonal fruits as you can. Substitute wholemeal flour for white flour in all your recipes and avoid those that include a large amount of syrup, sugar or treacle. The cookery books you already have will contain plenty of ideas for cooking vegetables and making interesting salads, but I have made a few suggestions for some main meal salads, some using brown rice.

I hope you'll enjoy trying out these recipes and developing your own ideas and adaptations. You are most likely to be successful in changing your family's eating habits if you do it gradually, trying out one or two new things a week. Happy cooking!

Soups

A bowl of home-made soup with croutons or some wholemeal bread, followed by cheese and fruit, makes a delicious and satisfying meal which is easy to prepare. Many soups are based on a meat stock, but nowadays few housewives keep a traditional stockpot or even a bowl of stock in the fridge because they usually buy small joints of meat which only give small amounts of stock, and few supermarkets have bones for sale. But you can ask your butcher for them or if you cook a joint or a chicken use the bones for stock.

Meat stock

Meat bones
Bacon rinds
Onion
Carrot
Celery, mushrooms or leeks
Bay leaf, parsley, thyme or sage
Put the bones and bacon rinds into a large pan, cover with cold water and add a coarsely chopped onion and carrot, celery, mushrooms or leeks and herbs. Bring to the boil and simmer gently for several hours or until reduced by one third. Strain into a large bowl and when cool put into the fridge. This stock will keep for several days in the fridge (otherwise it must be boiled up daily) and is very useful for soup, sauces and gravy.

When you boil a bacon joint keep the water as a stock for lentil or pea soup.

If you don't make your own stock, stock cubes are very useful but remember that they usually contain a lot of salt.
Croutons: Small cubes of wholemeal bread fried in butter until golden brown make a delicious garnish for many soups.

Basic vegetable mixture for soup

1 oz margarine, oil or dripping
1 onion
2 carrots
2 sticks celery

1 or 2 potatoes
2 rashers streaky bacon
Toss all these in the melted fat for 5 minutes. By adding other ingredients a variety of soups can be made.

Tomato soup

Basic vegetable mixture
1 15-oz can of tomatoes
1 pint stock or water
1 teaspoon oregano or basil
Wholemeal croutons
Add the tomatoes to the basic vegetable mixture then add the stock or water and the herbs. Simmer gently for 30 minutes. Pass through a sieve or liquidise, and serve garnished with croutons.

Split pea soup

Basic vegetable mixture
½ lb yellow or green split peas
3 pints stock, 'bacon water' or water
Chopped parsley
Add the peas to the basic vegetable mixture, then add the stock or water. Simmer for 1½ hours or until the peas are soft. Pass through a sieve or liquidise and add chopped parsley before serving.

Mixed vegetable soup

1 parsnip
1 leek
1 swede or turnip
Peas
Broad beans
Basic vegetable mixture
2 pints of stock or water
Salt and pepper
1 bayleaf
Chopped parsley or chives
Add the chopped vegetables to the vegetables in the basic vegetable mixture when making it, then add the stock or water,

seasoning and bayleaf. Simmer gently until the vegetables are tender. Pass through a sieve, liquidise or serve as it is. Add chopped parsley or chives before serving.

Lentil soup

8 oz lentils
Basic vegetable mixture
3 pints stock or water
1 teaspoon mixed herbs
Croutons
Add the lentils to the basic vegetable mixture, then add the stock or water and mixed herbs. Simmer for 1½ hours or until the vegetables are tender. Pass through a sieve or liquidise. Serve garnished with croutons.

Onion soup

4 large onions
2 rashers bacon
1 oz margarine
2 pints stock (or 2 pints water plus 2 stock cubes)
1 teaspoon mixed herbs or a bouquet garni
Chopped parsley
Salt and pepper (unless using stock cubes)
Gently cook the chopped bacon and sliced onion in the melted fat, then add the stock, herbs and seasoning and simmer gently for 30 minutes.

French onion soup

Onion soup as above
Slices of wholemeal bread
Cheddar, Parmesan or Gruyère cheese
Pour the readymade onion soup into a dish, lay the slices of bread on top, sprinkle with grated cheese and brown under the grill.

Mushroom soup

½ lb mushrooms
1 onion

1 potato
2 oz margarine
½ teaspoon dried thyme or 3 sprigs fresh thyme
2 pints stock
Salt and pepper
Chopped parsley
Slice mushrooms, onion and potato, and cook gently in melted margarine until the onion softens. Stir in thyme, then add stock and seasoning and simmer gently for 20 minutes. Add chopped parsley before serving.

Leek and potato soup

3 large leeks
1 lb potatoes
1 oz margarine or dripping
1½ pints stock or water
½ cup milk or cream
Salt and pepper
Chopped parsley
Finely slice the leeks and potatoes, making sure you retain some of the green part of the leeks to give the soup a good colour. Cook the vegetables gently in the melted fat until soft but not coloured. Add stock and seasoning and simmer for 30 minutes. Pass through a sieve or liquidise, then reheat gently without boiling and stir in the milk or cream. Add chopped parsley before serving.

Meat dishes

Hamburgers

1 lb minced beef
1 onion
1 egg
3 tablespoons quick-cooking oats (or 3 tablespoons oatmeal soaked in 3 tablespoons hot water for 30 minutes)
½ teaspoon dried mixed herbs
Salt and pepper
Worcester sauce
Mix the meat with the finely chopped onion, then add the egg,

oats, herbs, seasoning and Worcester sauce. Mix well and shape into rounds. This amount should make 8 medium-sized hamburgers. Fry in shallow fat, grill or barbecue.

Meat loaf

1 onion
1 carrot
½ green pepper
1 lb minced beef
1 egg
3–4 tablespoons quick-cooking porridge oats (or oatmeal or wholemeal breadcrumbs)
Salt and pepper
Mixed herbs to taste
Tomato puree or ketchup

Finely chop the onion, carrot and pepper, then mix all the ingredients together except for the tomato puree. Season well and put into an ovenproof dish or loaf tin. Cover the surface with a layer of tomato puree and cook in a moderate oven (375°F or Gas No 5) for 1 hour.

Moussaka

3 aubergines
1–1½ lb boneless lamb
1 oz fat
2 onions
1 large can of tomatoes or 1 lb fresh tomatoes
Oregano
Salt and pepper
Cheese sauce: Make a cheese sauce using ¾ pint of milk and thickening with wholemeal flour.

Cut the aubergines into ¼-inch slices. Sprinkle with salt and leave for half an hour. Drain thoroughly. Cook sliced onions and chopped lamb in melted fat until lightly browned. Put a layer of this mixture into a deep casserole and cover with a layer of aubergines, then a layer of sliced tomatoes. Season each layer and sprinkle the oregano on to the tomatoes. Repeat the layers and then cover with the cheese sauce.

Cook in a moderate oven (375°F or Gas No 5) for 1 hour with the lid on, then remove lid and cook for a further 45 minutes or until the cheese is lightly browned. This dish can be kept hot in a low oven for a long time and is useful if guests may be late.

A layer of sliced potatoes between the aubergines and tomatoes makes a complete meal for the family.

Stuffed shoulder of lamb

1 whole or half shoulder of lamb
Oatmeal stuffing (see section on oatmeal below)
Rosemary
Bone the shoulder if you can or ask the butcher to do it for you. Put the oatmeal stuffing into the cavity where the bone was. Make the meat into as neat a roll as you can and tie with string in several places. Put into a roasting tin with some fresh rosemary (or sprinkle with dried rosemary). Roast in a hot oven (420°F or Gas No 7) for 20 minutes per lb and 20 minutes over.

Macaroni cheese with vegetables

8 oz wholemeal macaroni
Mixed vegetables (e.g. onions, carrots, celery, mushrooms, sweet corn)
Margarine or oil
1 pint cheese sauce
2 tomatoes (optional)
2 tablespoons breadcrumbs
Cook wholemeal macaroni as directed on packet. Drain and rinse quickly under cold tap. Cook mixed vegetables gently in margarine or oil and mix with the macaroni. Stir in the cheese sauce and put the mixture into a shallow dish. Cover with thinly sliced tomatoes and sprinkle with breadcrumbs and grated cheese. Brown under the grill.

Stew and dumplings
Stew

2 onions
Margarine or oil

1½ lb stewing beef
1 oz wholemeal flour
Mixed herbs
1 carrot
2 tomatoes
Salt and pepper
Water or stock to cover (or half-and-half red wine and stock)

Slice the onions, brown in the fat and put aside. Trim the beef and cut into cubes, brown in the fat, then sprinkle with the flour and herbs and stir well. Add the onions, sliced carrot, coarsely chopped tomatoes and seasoning. Stir in the water, stock or wine plus stock. Cook in a deep casserole for 1½–2 hours at 325°F or Gas No 2.

Dumplings

4 oz wholemeal flour
2 teaspoons baking powder
2 oz shredded suet
½ teaspoon salt
Pepper
1 tablespoon chopped parsley
2–3 tablespoons water

Mix flour, baking powder, suet, seasoning and parsley. Add 2–3 tablespoons cold water to mix. Form into small balls and put on top of the stew to cook for 30 minutes before serving.

Brown rice

Brown rice is available in all health food shops, many supermarkets and in specialist shops selling grains, beans and flour. It's very different from the white rice that most people are used to eating. It takes about 40–50 minutes to cook in boiling salted water and has a chewy texture. It is delicious hot or cold and is more filling than white rice so you'll need less per person.

IDEAS FOR USING RICE IN SAVOURY DISHES:

8 oz brown rice cooked in plenty of boiling salted water should be enough for 4 people.

Fish with rice

8 oz brown rice (cooked)
12 oz cooked smoked fish (or an 8 oz tin of tuna or salmon)
1–2 hardboiled eggs
Parsley
Butter
Coarsely chop the eggs and mix all the ingredients together.
Serve very hot.

Vegetables with rice

8 oz brown rice (cooked)
1 carrot
1 pepper
¼ lb mushrooms
A few peas
Margarine or oil
2–4 oz grated cheese
Salt and pepper
Chop the vegetables and cook in melted fat, then stir into the
cooked rice. Mix well, season and serve sprinkled with grated
cheese.

A few rashers of streaky bacon chopped into small pieces can
be cooked with the vegetables if desired; similarly left over
ham or the end of a joint of beef, pork or lamb can be finely
chopped and mixed with the vegetables to heat through before
adding to the rice. If you add meat you will not need to serve
grated cheese as well.

Stuffed marrow

1 onion
4 oz cooked meat or 4 oz mince
Margarine or oil
2 cups cooked brown rice (or 1 cup cooked rice and 1 cup
wholemeal breadcrumbs)
Parsley
2 tomatoes
Salt and pepper
1 medium sized marrow

Gently cook the chopped onion and meat in margarine or oil for 10 minutes, then add the rice and chopped parsley. Stir the coarsely chopped tomatoes into the rice mixture and season.

Peel the marrow and slice lengthways so that you have a thin slice and a thick one. Scoop out the seeds and fill the boat-shaped thicker slice with the stuffing. Place the thinner 'lid' on top, and tie in several places with string. Season and dot with butter. Place in a greased tin and bake for 1–1½ hours or until tender at 350°F or Gas No 4. Alternatively the marrow can be left with the skin on and cut into slices 1 inch thick. Remove the seeds and put into a greased tin. Fill with stuffing and bake for about 30 minutes or until tender at 350°F or Gas No 4.

This dish is good if served with cheese sauce.

Stuffed peppers

1 onion
2 oz bacon or ham
4 oz mushrooms
Margarine or oil
1 cup cooked brown rice
Salt and pepper
4 large peppers

Cook the chopped onion, bacon and mushrooms gently in margarine or oil for 10 minutes. Add the cooked rice and season. Cut the tops off the peppers and remove the seeds. Cook in boiling water for 3 minutes and drain. Fill the peppers with the stuffing, replace the tops and put into a baking dish with a little water. Bake for about 30–35 minutes or until soft at 375°F or Gas No 5.

Stuffed tomatoes

Tomatoes may be stuffed and cooked in the same way as peppers.

Stuffed cabbage leaves

2 young cabbage leaves per person
3 spring onions or 1 small onion
¼ lb mushrooms

Butter
4 oz cooked meat or ham (optional)
Salt and pepper
Fresh or dried mixed herbs to taste
1 cup cooked rice or wholemeal breadcrumbs
1 cup stock
Cook cabbage leaves in boiling salted water for 5 minutes to soften them. Cook the sliced onions and mushrooms in butter for 5 minutes, then add the finely chopped meat or ham. Add the seasoning, herbs and rice and mix well. Place each cabbage leaf flat and put about a tablespoon of filling at the base of each leaf. Fold over and form into neat parcels, tying with string. Put into a shallow dish and add the stock. Bring to the boil and cover, then cook for 10–15 minutes or until tender.

Vegetables

Potatoes

Here are a few recipes for potatoes which make them a delicious vegetable instead of the rather boring, white, insipid objects most people think they are.

Boiled potatoes

Always boil potatoes in their skins, having scrubbed them and removed any blemishes first. Boil in salted water until soft and then drain. Leaving them to dry out in an ovenproof dish in a warm oven for 10 minutes or more will improve the flavour a lot.

Roast potatoes

Roast potatoes in their skins, having scrubbed them and removed any blemishes first. Roast in the fat round the joint in the oven.

Potatoes dauphinoise

1½ lb potatoes
¾ pint creamy milk (½ pint milk plus ¼ pint single cream)
Salt and pepper
Garlic

Scrub the potatoes and slice thinly. Rinse with cold water and dry in a clean tea towel. Rub a shallow ovenproof dish with garlic and then butter. Fill with potatoes, seasoning each layer. Pour the milk over the potatoes so that they are just covered, dot with butter and bake at 325°F or Gas No 3 for 1–2 hours until cooked and nicely browned. This is a dish that keeps well in the oven and is delicious with hot or cold meat.

Potato casserole

1½ lb potatoes
2 medium sized onions
Salt and pepper

Cheese sauce:

1 oz butter
1 oz wholemeal flour
½ pint milk
4–6 oz grated cheese
Salt and pepper
Scrub the potatoes and cut into thin slices. Slice the onions. Fill a greased casserole dish with potatoes and onions in layers, finishing with potato. Season.

Make the cheese sauce in your usual way, reserving 1 oz of cheese for topping. Pour the sauce over the vegetables and sprinkle the remaining cheese on top. Cook in a moderate oven (400°F or Gas No 6) for 1–1½ hours or until the dish is cooked.

This is delicious with a cabbage salad.

Pan hagerty

1 lb potatoes
½ lb onions
1 oz fat
4–6 oz grated cheese
Salt and pepper
Scrub the potatoes and cut into thin slices. Slice the onions. Heat the fat in a frying pan and put in layers of potato, onion, cheese, seasoning, potato, onion and potato again, finishing with a layer of cheese. Cover the pan and cook for 15–20

minutes. Brown the top under the grill and serve. For a more substantial dish add some chopped bacon and sliced tomatoes to the onion layer.

Cabbage

Cabbage casserole

1–2 lb cabbage
½ lb tomatoes (or 1 small tin of tomatoes)
Sausage ring (or garlic sausage, cooked ham or bacon)
White sauce (made with 1 oz wholemeal flour, 1 oz butter, ½ pint milk)
2 oz grated cheese
2 tablespoons wholemeal breadcrumbs

Boil the cabbage in a little salted water until tender. Butter an ovenproof dish and put a layer of cabbage into the bottom.
Cover with a layer of tomatoes and a few slices of a sausage ring or other meat. Cover with another layer of cabbage and top with white sauce. Sprinkle with breadcrumbs and grated cheese. Bake at 375°F or Gas No 5 for 40 minutes until brown. N.B. Mushrooms may be used instead of meat. This dish goes well with baked potatoes.

Salads

Raw vegetables and salads provide a lot of fibre and are easy to prepare. There is no need to make a complicated mixture – just slice up some cucumber, cut a carrot and some celery into sticks and put them on a plate beside your bread and cheese or cold meat, or pop them into a plastic bag for your sandwich lunch or picnic. Here are a few recipes and ideas to help you start. You'll soon find favourites of your own.

Substantial salads

suitable for a main dish to be served with potatoes or bread

Cabbage salad

1 small white cabbage (about 1–1½ lb)
3 tablespoons oil

1½ tablespoons vinegar
1 carrot
1 eating apple
2 spring onions (or 1 tablespoon chopped chives)
2 sticks celery
½–1 green pepper
cucumber (2–3 in.)
1 tomato
2 oz raisins or chopped dates
2–4 oz cashew nuts
Salt and pepper
Chop the cabbage finely, rinse in cold water and drain well. Add the oil, vinegar, scrubbed grated carrot, apple grated in its skin, finely chopped onions, chopped celery, pepper, cucumber and tomato and mix well. Stir in the raisins and cashew nuts and season before serving. This forms a substantial salad and is delicious with baked potatoes in their jackets.

The nuts and dates can be omitted and chopped ham or small cubes of cheese added instead.

Rice salad

3 cups cooked brown rice
4 tablespoons oil
2 tablespoons vinegar
Salt and pepper
1–2 tomatoes
1–2 spring onions
1 green pepper
2 sticks celery
Drain the rice, rinse with hot water and cool. Add oil, vinegar and seasoning and mix well. Stir in chopped tomatoes and onions, sliced pepper and celery.

This rice salad may be combined with any of the following:

1 Pickled herring and onion plus 2 tablespoons yoghourt or cream
2 1 8-oz can salmon, 2 chopped hardboiled eggs and some chopped parsley

3 I 8-oz can tuna, 2–3 gherkins and I tablespoon mayonnaise
4 I cup chopped cold chicken and I red dessert apple chopped
in its skin.

These rice salads make very good and easy picnics – serve them
in plastic bowls and eat with a spoon.

Chicken and chicory salad

12 oz cooked chicken
3 sticks celery
2 pieces chicory
I green pepper
2 tablespoons salad cream
2 tablespoons cream
Salt and pepper
I tablespoon fresh tarragon (optional)
Chop the chicken, vegetables and tarragon and mix all the
ingredients together. Chill and serve with lettuce or tomato rice
salad.

Cheese and apple salad

6–8 oz Cheddar or Dutch cheese
2 large eating apples
3 sticks celery
2 tablespoons chopped dates
2 gherkins (optional)
4 tablespoons oil
2 tablespoons vinegar
Salt and pepper
Chop the cheese, apples, celery and gherkins and mix all the
ingredients together. Serve with a lettuce or cabbage salad.

Tuna salad

I can tuna
I onion
2–3 sticks celery
I pepper
Cucumber (2–3 in.)

3 tablespoons mayonnaise
1 tablespoon lemon juice
1 tablespoon capers or chopped gherkin
Salt and pepper

Drain the oil from the tuna and flake the fish. Chop the onion, celery, pepper and cucumber and mix all the ingredients together. Chill and serve with lettuce leaves.

Other lighter salads
Simple cabbage salad

1 lb white cabbage
1 carrot
1 dessert apple
2 tablespoons oil
1–2 tablespoons vinegar
1–2 tablespoons yoghourt
Salt and pepper

Grate the cabbage, scrubbed carrot and apple in its skin. Mix all the ingredients together.

Beetroot and bean salad

2 cups cooked beetroot
1 onion
1 cup cooked butter beans
1 cup cooked French beans
Oil and vinegar dressing
Salt and pepper

Coarsely chop the beetroot and thinly slice the onion. Mix all the ingredients together and chill.

Tomato rice salad

2 cups cooked brown rice
Oil and vinegar dressing
3 large tomatoes
1 onion (optional)
Salt and pepper
Fresh basil or thyme

Stir the dressing into the cooled rice. Add the sliced tomatoes, finely chopped onion and seasoning. Sprinkle with finely chopped basil or thyme and chill for an hour for the flavours to blend.

Potato salad

1½ lb potatoes
1 tablespoon finely chopped onion or chives
1 tablespoon chopped parsley
2 tablespoons mayonnaise
2 tablespoons oil and vinegar dressing
Salt and pepper
Garlic to taste

Scrub the potatoes and cook in their skins in boiling salted water. Drain and coarsely chop. Mix all the ingredients together and serve hot or cold with meat or sausage.

Other simple salads can be made by slicing up vegetables and tossing them in an oil and vinegar dressing, then adding onion, garlic or herbs to taste:

1 Grated carrot and apple
2 Sliced tomatoes, sliced onions and basil or marjoram
3 Sliced, cooked beetroot and watercress
4 French beans and chopped onions
5 Sliced green and red peppers
6 Cucumber and green peppers
7 Shredded or grated Kohlrabi
8 Chicory and tomato
9 Celery and apple or celery and date
10 Sliced button mushrooms

Cold stuffed tomatoes

1 large tomato or 2 smaller ones per person
4 tablespoons wholemeal breadcrumbs
1 8-oz can pilchards in tomato sauce
1 chopped spring onion or 1 teaspoon chopped chives
1 tablespoon chopped parsley
1 tablespoon vinegar or lemon juice
2 tablespoons oil
Salt and pepper

Stand the tomatoes upside down and cut the tops off them. Scoop out the insides with a spoon or sharply pointed knife and drain. Mash the tomato pulp, juice and seeds, and stir in the breadcrumbs. Mix in the mashed pilchards, onion, parsley, vinegar, oil and seasoning. Fill tomatoes with the mixture and replace the lids. Serve with a green salad or other salad vegetable.

Beans and lentils

In these days of soaring meat prices, it is a help to have some recipes which only require a small quantity of it. Beans and lentils are high in protein and make a very good meat-stretching meal.

Haricot mutton

1 onion
1 oz dripping
1 lb lean mutton
1 pint stock or water
Salt and pepper
½ lb parboiled haricot beans
1 carrot
1 turnip

Slice the onion, brown in the fat and put aside. Trim the meat, cut into chunks and brown in the fat. Add the stock or water and seasoning, bring to the boil and skim. Add beans and onions, stir well and simmer slowly for 1 hour. Add diced carrot and turnip and cook until tender.

Butter beans in sauce

1 lb butter beans, soaked overnight
¼ lb bacon
1 onion
1 lb tomatoes (tinned or fresh)
1 teaspoon chilli powder
1 teaspoon salt
1½ pints stock or water

Cover the beans and sliced bacon with the sliced onion and chopped tomato in an ovenproof dish. Sprinkle with chilli powder and salt. Pour over the stock and bake slowly for about 2 hours at 325°F or Gas No 3.

Bean pot (serves 8–12)

2 large onions
1–2 garlic cloves
12 oz belly pork
1 oz dripping
1½ lb assorted beans (e.g. haricot, blackeyed, red, black, butter, soaked overnight)
Oregano
1 small tin tomato puree (optional)
2 stock cubes
Fry the sliced onions, crushed or chopped garlic and chopped pork in the dripping until lightly browned. Put the beans in a separate pan, cover with water and bring to the boil. Discard the water and repeat 3 times. This process helps to make the beans more digestible. Stir the drained beans into the pork and onion mixture and cover with water to 1 inch over the top. Stir in the oregano, stock cubes and tomato puree. Bring to the boil then cook in a slow oven (275–300°F or Gas No 1) for 4–6 hours. Check that the beans do not become dry.

Serve with baked potatoes in their jackets.
NB Instead of belly pork you can use a bacon hock, a piece of bacon flank, bacon scraps or ½–1 lb minced beef.

This dish keeps well in the fridge for several days and can be reheated. Leftovers can be liquidised with some water to make a thick and satisfying soup.

Haricot beans with onions and tomatoes

½ lb haricot beans, soaked overnight and cooked until tender
1 large onion
Margarine
2–3 tomatoes
Pinch of mixed herbs
Salt and pepper

Cook the chopped onion in margarine until soft. Add the peeled and chopped tomatoes, mixed herbs and seasoning. Simmer for 5 minutes then stir in cooked beans very gently. Serve hot with meat or sausage.

Lentils

1 lb green or brown lentils
1 onion
1 clove garlic
Oil or dripping
Stock or water to cover
1 teaspoon mixed herbs
Salt and pepper

Look over the lentils and pick out any pieces of grit. Fry the onion and crushed or chopped garlic gently in the dripping for 5 minutes, and then stir in the lentils, herbs and seasoning. Cover with plenty of stock or water to 1 inch over the top of the lentils, and bring to the boil. Simmer very gently for approximately 1 hour or until the lentils are soft, or put into a casserole and cook in a slow oven (275–300°F or Gas No 1) for 1½–2 hours. If the liquid dries up before the lentils are soft, add some more boiling water.

These lentils are delicious eaten on their own with a generous pat of butter.

Lentils and bacon

1–2 lb bacon joint, fat or lean
1 onion
1 carrot
1 stick celery
1 garlic clove
Oil or dripping
1 teaspoon mixed herbs
1 lb brown or green lentils

Cover the bacon joint with cold water, bring to the boil and drain. Cook the chopped onion, carrot, celery and garlic gently for 5 minutes in the dripping. Add the herbs and lentils and stir well. Put the bacon joint into a deep casserole and add the lentils and vegetables. Cover with cold water, bring to the boil and cook slowly for 2 hours or until the lentils are soft.

Pizza, pancakes and fritters

Pizza dough

1 lb wholemeal flour
2 level teaspoons salt
½ oz dried yeast
1 teaspoon sugar
1 tablespoon oil
Approx. ½ pint water

Put the flour and salt into a large bowl. Mix the yeast and sugar and add ¼ pint warm water, mix well with a fork and leave in a warm place for 10 minutes. Add the oil to the yeast liquid, pour into a well in the flour and mix to a soft dough using the rest of the warm water. Knead until smooth and leave in a warm place for 40 minutes or until double in size. Knead again lightly, divide into portions if you wish to make small pizzas, or press into a flat baking tin for a large one. Press the dough out to fit the well-greased tins and leave for 10 minutes. Add the topping of your choice and bake in a hot oven (450°F or Gas No 8) for 20–25 minutes.

Pizza sauce

1 large onion
1–2 sticks celery
Oil or dripping
1 green pepper
1 tin tomatoes (15 oz)
1 teaspoon oregano or basil
Salt and pepper
1 clove garlic
6 oz Cheddar cheese

Cook the coarsely chopped onion, garlic and celery gently in the fat for 10 minutes, then add the coarsely chopped green pepper and toss it in the fat. Stir in the chopped tomatoes, herbs and seasoning. Cook very gently for 20 minutes and cool before using. This sauce can be made while the pizza dough is rising. Spread on to the pizza base, sprinkle the grated cheese evenly over the top and bake in a hot oven (450°F or Gas No 8) for 20–25 minutes.

For a different pizza you can add other ingredients, placing them on top of the pizza sauce in a pattern and then sprinkling with cheese.

Suggested toppings for pizza

1 Black olives and anchovy fillets
2 Sardines
3 Salami slices
4 Add bacon cut up in small pieces to the pizza sauce when you are cooking the celery and onion
5 Other cheese can be used such as Gruyère or Cheshire
6 Cold ham or cooked bacon.

Pancake batter

4 oz wholemeal flour
Pinch salt
1 egg
1 tablespoon oil
½ pint milk (or milk and water)
Put the flour and salt into a basin. Add the egg and oil and beat well. Gradually add the liquid to make a smooth batter. If you do this slowly you are less likely to get lumps. Allow to stand for at least 30 minutes before use, preferably in the fridge. Beat again before use.
To cook pancakes: Heat a small quantity of butter or margarine in a frying pan, and when hot pour in a little of the batter. Fill the pan so that the batter is evenly distributed. Turn over or toss when the surface is dull and cook until lightly browned on the other side. Turn on to greaseproof paper and keep warm.

This quantity of batter will make about 12 pancakes. They can be placed in a pile, covered with greaseproof paper and kept warm until being filled before serving. Alternatively they can be filled and reheated later.

Suggested fillings
Savoury

1 Tinned asparagus
2 Mushroom, tomato and onion, or pepper, onion and tomato cooked gently in butter.
3 Place the pancakes one on top of the other, sprinkling each with grated cheese and layering with thinly sliced tomatoes. Top with grated cheese and heat through in the oven. Serve in wedges.
4 Tuna and hard boiled egg covered with white sauce (made with wholemeal flour), sprinkled with grated cheese and browned under the grill.
5 Chopped ham in cheese sauce
6 Shrimps and mushrooms in white sauce (made with wholemeal flour)
7 Mushroom, bacon and onion cooked gently in butter, plus cheese sauce.
NB Recipes 5, 6 and 7 are very good as the first course for dinner parties if the sauce is poured over the filled pancakes instead of being used in the filling. They can be kept in the oven before serving.

Sweet

1 Apple puree or stewed apple
2 Sliced banana tossed in lemon juice
3 Stewed fruit (e.g. blackcurrants or gooseberries)

Yorkshire pudding

Use the basic pancake recipe. Heat some fat until smoking in a shallow tin, add the batter and cook in the top of a hot oven (425°F or Gas No 7) for 20–30 minutes or until well risen and brown.

Corn fritters

Basic pancake batter recipe, with only ¼ pint of the liquid
1 small can sweetcorn or 4 oz frozen sweetcorn
Oil or dripping

Stir the sweetcorn into the stiff pancake batter and mix well. Melt the fat and when hot put in a spoonful of the mixture. Cook until brown. Turn and cook the other side. Keep hot in a warm oven. These are delicious on their own or served with cold meat and salad. Children love them.
NB Flaked tuna fish can be added and the fritters cooked in the same way.

Vegetable fritters

Basic pancake batter recipe with only $\frac{1}{4}$ pint of the liquid
Vegetables (whole or sliced), lightly cooked (boiled or steamed)
Fat or oil
Dip the vegetables in the stiff batter and fry in hot fat (deep or shallow) until brown. Sprinkle very lightly with salt and pepper and keep warm in the oven.
NB Parsnips and Jerusalem artichokes are good for this dish, as are raw aubergines.

Sweet fritters

Basic pancake batter recipe with only $\frac{1}{4}$ pint of the liquid
Fruit (e.g. cooking apples peeled [optional], cored and sliced in rings, sliced banana, pineapple rings)
Oil
Dip the fruit in the stiff batter and fry in hot fat (deep or shallow) until brown. Sprinkle lightly with sugar and keep warm in the oven.

Ways with oatmeal
Fried herring or mackerel in oatmeal

4 fish
2 tablespoons medium-grade oatmeal
Salt and pepper
Oil or dripping
Parsley and lemon
Clean and fillet fish, mix oatmeal and seasoning and toss the fish in it. Cook the fish in heated fat until brown on both sides. Serve garnished with parsley and lemon.

Oatcakes

4 oz medium oatmeal
½ teaspoon salt
1–2 teaspoons melted dripping
Pinch of bicarbonate of soda
Warm water

Slowly heat griddle. Mix oatmeal, salt, dripping and soda to a soft consistency with warm water. Turn on to a board sprinkled with dry oatmeal and knead well. Form into rounds and roll out as thinly as possible without cracking. Cut rounds into 4 or 8 wedges, and bake until the edges curl up. Toast in front of the fire or place for a few minutes in a hot oven to dry. Cool and keep in an airtight tin.

These can be baked in the oven at 325°F or Gas No 3 for 15–20 minutes if you haven't got a griddle.

Oatmeal stuffing 1

1 small onion
1 teaspoon parsley
4 oz medium oatmeal
2 oz chopped suet
Salt and pepper
Stock

Chop the onion and the parsley. Mix all the ingredients, moistening with the stock. Use for stuffing a boiling fowl.

Oatmeal stuffing 2

1 onion
1 oz margarine or dripping
2 rashers streaky bacon
3–4 mushrooms
1–2 sticks celery (optional)
2–3 oz medium oatmeal
Salt and pepper
Thyme and parsley
Grated lemon rind

Finely chop the onion and bacon and fry gently in the fat for 5 minutes. Chop the mushrooms and celery, add to the pan, mix well and fry gently for a further 5 minutes. Stir in the oatmeal, seasoning, herbs and lemon rind. Use for stuffing a roasting chicken.

NB 3 or 4 crushed juniper berries add an unusual flavour to the stuffing. If the chicken has giblets, chop the liver and fry with the bacon and vegetables. Any stuffing which is left over in the chicken helps to flavour the stock you make with the chicken bones, but use this stock as soon as possible because the stuffing doesn't keep very well.

Porridge

Porridge made with oatmeal is really delicious, particularly if eaten with salt and not covered with sugar or syrup.

4 oz fine or medium oatmeal
2 pints water
Salt to taste

Bring water to the boil, add salt and oatmeal. Simmer gently for 30 minutes, stirring occasionally. It's a good idea to do this in a double saucepan if you have one. Serve with milk and salt to taste.

Puddings with fruit

Stewed fruit

This is useful for an easy pudding, served with cream or topped with crisp cereal. Adding finely sliced cooking apples to gooseberries, rhubarb or blackcurrants takes away some of the acidity, and so less sugar is needed. Fresh apricots are delicious stewed with a dessertspoon of vanilla essence per 1 lb of fruit. When you cook dried fruit do not add extra sugar – add a few strips of grated lemon peel for flavour.

Fresh fruit puddings

1 Fresh fruit salad. Use orange juice instead of syrup
2 Thinly sliced oranges with a tablespoon of liqueur such as Cointreau
3 Melon
4 Fresh pineapple
5 Melon cut into cubes and mixed with 1 or 2 pieces of finely

chopped stem ginger. Serve well chilled. Fresh pears are also delicious served in this way. Prevent the fruit from browning by tossing it in 1 teaspoon lemon juice plus 2 tablespoons water

Ideas for yoghourt and fruit

Buy natural unsweetened yoghourt and add fruit yourself.
1 Add an orange cut into small pieces
2 Mash some bananas (ideal for the cheaper ones which are brown and over-ripe) and mix with juice of 1 orange. Stir in yoghourt
3 Chop left-over stewed prunes (or liquidise them) and add to yoghourt
4 Cooked mixed dried fruit salad is delicious with yoghourt
5 Mash strawberries, raspberries or loganberries and add some sugar to taste, then mix with yoghourt
6 Add stewed gooseberries or blackcurrants

Crisp flan case with fruit filling

2 oz margarine
1 tablespoon honey
2 oz wholewheat flakes or bran flakes
Melt margarine and stir in the honey. Add the flakes and mix well. Press into a shallow dish and leave until firm – this can be hastened by putting into the fridge. This flan case can then be filled with a variety of fruit mixtures.

Crispy blackcurrant flan

1 flan case
$\frac{1}{2}$ lb blackcurrants
2 tablespoons sugar
Wholemeal flour
2 eggs
Stew blackcurrants with sugar. Thicken with flour (1 tablespoon mixed with 2 tablespoons water will be plenty), and pour into the flan.

This can be made more special by beating 2 egg yolks into the thickened puree and folding in the well beaten egg whites. Chill and serve with single or whipped cream.

Crispy gooseberry flan

Use the recipe for Crispy blackcurrant flan but substitute ½ lb gooseberries.

Hot puddings with fruit:
Fruit crumbles

These are easy to make and always popular. They can be made with fruit which has already been stewed or with fresh fruit with a small quantity of sugar and water. Cover with basic crumble mix and bake in a moderate oven (375°F or Gas No 5) for 30–40 minutes or until fruit is soft.

Apples, apple and blackberries, rhubarb, gooseberries and plums are all good cooked this way.

Basic crumble mix

8 oz wholemeal flour
4 oz margarine or cooking fat
1 teaspoon sugar

Crunchy oat topping for stewed fruit (such as rhubarb, apples, gooseberries)

2 oz margarine or butter
6 tablespoons quick cooking porridge oats
1 teaspoon sugar
1 teaspoon spice (optional)

Melt fat and add oats, sugar and spice of your choice. Mix well, sprinkle on to the fruit and bake in a hot oven (400°F or Gas No 6) for 30 minutes or until the top is light brown.

NB Instead of adding 6 tablespoons of oats you can add 3 tablespoons of wholemeal breadcrumbs and 3 tablespoons of oats mixed together.

Gooseberry crunch

1 lb gooseberries
Sugar
2 oz margarine

1 tablespoon honey
2 cups wheat or bran flakes
Put fruit in a pie dish with a little water and add sugar to aste.
Melt margarine and honey and stir in the flakes. Pile the mix-
ture on to the fruit and bake in a moderate oven (375°F or
Gas No 5) until the fruit is cooked.

Apple Betty

2 oz butter or margarine
1½ cups wholemeal breadcrumbs
1 teaspoon cinnamon or cardamon
1½ lb cooking apples, pureed (see recipe, below)
Melt butter and add breadcrumbs. Stir well and allow to
brown lightly. Stir in the spice. Put a layer of this mixture into
a buttered baking dish, then a layer of apple and so on until
you have 3 layers of breadcrumbs and 2 layers of apples.

Dot with butter and bake in a hot oven (400°F or Gas No 6)
for 30 minutes. Serve with cream.

Baked apples

1 cooking apple per person
Sultanas, mincemeat or mixed dried fruit, 1 teaspoon for each
apple
Mixed spice to taste
Juice of an orange or some tinned pineapple juice
Butter or margarine
Wash and core the apples and score around the middles to
prevent them bursting while cooking. Put into a shallow pie
dish. Mix the fruit with the spice and use to stuff the centre of
each apple. Put a small quantity of margarine or butter on top
and pour the orange juice and an equal quantity of water into
the pie dish. Bake at 400°F or Gas No 6 for 45–60 minutes or
until apples are tender.

Blackberry and apple dumpling

Suet pastry	Fruit
8 oz wholemeal flour	1 lb apples (sliced)
Pinch salt	½ lb blackberries

3 oz shredded suet   1 teaspoon sugar
2 teaspoons baking powder
Water to mix

Mix flour, salt, suet and baking powder. Add water to make a soft dough. Roll out thinly and line a greased pudding basin with half the pastry. Fill with fruit and sugar and cover with remaining pastry. Steam or boil for 2–3 hours.

Basic apple puree:

1 lb cooking apples
3 tablespoons water
Sugar to taste

Wash, core and cook the apples with the water until soft. When cool press through a sieve or mouli, or liquidise. This produces a delicious apple puree and you can add sugar to taste. As you get used to eating non-sweet foods you will eventually find you don't want to add any sugar at all, particularly with ripe Bramleys.

A mixture of cooking and eating apples can be used, but eating apples alone do not have so much flavour when cooked. This puree can be kept in the fridge in a jar or covered container for up to a week, and is very useful for a variety of desserts.

Apple flan

Pastry flan case (see page 228)
Apple puree
Cinnamon, cardamon or allspice
1 eating apple
Butter
Sugar

Cover the uncooked flan case with apple puree. Sprinkle with spice. Thinly slice a washed and cored eating apple and arrange the slices in a pattern on top of the puree. Dot with butter and sprinkle very lighly with sugar though you may find it sweet enough without extra sugar. Bake at 425°F or Gas No 7 for 35–40 minutes.

Apricot and apple flan

Pastry flan case (see page 228)
Apple puree
Apricots, fresh or dried
Cover uncooked flan case with apple puree and cover with fresh apricot halves (or dried apricots which have been soaked and partly cooked in water). Cover with a lattice of pastry and bake in a hot oven (425°F or Gas No 7) for 35–40 minutes.

Blackcurrant flan

Pastry flan case (see page 228)
Blackcurrants
Wholemeal flour
Cook the flan case (for 10 minutes at 450°F or Gas No 8) filled with beans in greaseproof paper, then remove these and cook for a further 15–20 minutes or until crisp and golden. Fill with stewed blackcurrants thickened with flour. Serve hot or cold.

Strawberry flan

Pastry flan case (see page 228)
Strawberries
Sugar
Cream
Cook the flan case (see above recipe) and fill when cold with sliced strawberries. Sprinkle with sugar and decorate with whipped cream.

Mincemeat and apple flan

Pastry flan case (see page 228)
Mincemeat
Apples (cooking or dessert)
Partially cook the flan case (weighted with beans or peas in greaseproof paper for 10 minutes at 450 °F or Gas No 8) then fill with mincemeat and thinly sliced apples. Finish cooking at 425°F or Gas No 7 for 20–30 minutes. Serve hot or cold.

Fruit tart

Basic pastry recipe (see page 227)
Fruit (e.g. apple and blackberry; apple with cloves; apple and apricot; apple and dried fruit; apples, prunes [cooked and stoned] and spice; gooseberry; rhubarb; plums and cinnamon).
Milk or egg
Sugar
Line a greased ovenproof dish or shallow tin with half the pastry. Put in fruit filling and cover with remaining pastry. Prick with a fork and brush with milk or beaten egg. Sprinkle lightly with sugar. Bake at 425°F or Gas No 7 for 30 minutes or until nicely browned.
NB Sugar may be added to the filling if desired.

Fruit slices

Basic pastry recipe (see page 227)
Fruit e.g.:
1 Apple and sultanas
2 Dates soaked for 10 minutes in a small amount of boiling water to soften, and mixed with chopped walnuts
3 Dried apricots, soaked or boiled for 15–20 minutes
4 Dried figs, chopped and soaked in boiling water until soft.
Beaten egg or milk
Roll pastry into an oblong and cover half with one of the fillings. Fold the uncovered pastry over the fruit and seal the edges with water. Roll out lightly, cut into slices, brush with beaten egg or milk, prick with a fork and bake at 425°F or Gas No 7 for 20–30 minutes.

Apple balls

Basic pastry recipe (see page 227)
4 apples
Cloves
Sugar
Raisins, sultanas or dates
Beaten egg or milk
Divide pastry into 4 equal pieces, form into rounds and place a

cored apple on each. Fill each apple with either a clove and a teaspoon of sugar or some raisins, sultanas or dates.

Bring the pastry up over the apple and seal well. Place upside down on a greased baking sheet, brush with beaten egg or milk and bake in a moderately hot oven (400°F or Gas No 6) for about 40 minutes. Serve hot or cold.

NB Pears can be cooked in the same way.

Rice pudding

2 oz brown rice
1½ pints milk
1 teaspoon sugar
½ oz butter or margarine
Grated nutmeg

Grease a pie dish. Wash the rice, put in the dish with the milk and sugar. Stir well. Sprinkle with nutmeg and dot with butter. Cook in a slow oven (325°F or Gas No 3) for 2–2½ hours. Stir once or twice during the first hour to prevent rice sticking to the bottom.

NB Instead of sugar you can add 2 oz raisins or sultanas, this makes a change and is delicious.

Pastry

Pastry made with wholemeal flour is delicious and can be used for a great variety of savoury and sweet recipes.

Basic pastry recipe

8 oz wholemeal flour
1 teaspoon salt
4 oz margarine or cooking fat
Water to mix

Mix the flour and salt and rub in the fat. Mix with water to a stiff and slightly wet dough and roll out lightly on a floured board. If you have time to let the dough rest for 30–60 minutes before use it is easier to roll out. Cook in a hot oven (425°F or Gas No 7).

Storage: The flour and fat mixture can be prepared without the water and stored in a sealed container in the fridge for several days until needed.

Add the water before using.

Leftover pastry can be stored for 1–2 days in the fridge.

Pastry flan case

Line a flan tin with pastry and put a piece of greaseproof paper inside, with a few beans or peas to weight it down. Cook for 10 minutes at 450°F or Gas No 8. Remove the paper and beans and the flan is ready to be filled before further baking.

Flan cases can be partly cooked like this, cooled and wrapped and then put in the freezer until needed. They form a very useful standby since they can be quickly filled with savoury or sweet fillings and baked to produce a delicious supper or dessert. (They can also be kept in the fridge or an airtight tin for several days – they are best wrapped in foil or polythene.)

Suggestions for savoury fillings for flan cases:

1 Fried chopped bacon, tomatoes and mixed herbs
2 Asparagus tips and grated cheese
3 Fried chopped mushrooms or whole baby mushrooms, plus thyme
4 Chopped cooked chicken and mushrooms
5 Thinly sliced tomatoes and grated cheese with parsley
6 Lightly cooked sliced onions and grated cheese
7 Prawns and lightly cooked mushrooms
8 Chopped spinach cooked with a finely chopped onion

Once you have put enough filling in the *partly cooked* flan case to cover its base, pour on an egg and milk mixture – 2 eggs beaten in ½ pint of milk with salt and pepper added. A sprinkling of fresh mixed herbs added to the egg mixture adds extra interest as does finely chopped parsley sprinkled on top of the cooked flan before serving. Bake for 20–30 minutes at 400°F or Gas No 6.

Alternatively flan cases can be *completely cooked* and then filled with cooked filling. To cook completely fill the case with beans in greaseproof paper to weight it for 10 minutes at 450°F or Gas No 8, then remove the beans and paper and cook for a further 15–20 minutes or until crisp and golden.

Suggestions for cooked fillings

1 Salmon in white sauce (made with wholemeal flour)
2 Cooked sliced onions and tomatoes topped with grated cheese and grilled
3 Mushrooms and onions in white sauce (made with wholemeal flour)
4 Cooked fish in white sauce (made with wholemeal flour, topped with grated cheese and browned under the grill.

Sausage rolls

Basic pastry recipe (see page 227)
½ lb sausage meat
1 onion or 1 dessertspoon chopped chives
Salt and pepper
Egg or milk
Mix the sausage meat, onion or chives and seasoning. Roll out the pastry and form into sausage rolls. Brush with beaten egg or milk and prick with a fork. Bake at 400°F or Gas No 6 for 20 minutes or until nicely browned.

Large sausage pie

Basic pastry recipe (see page 227)
1 lb sausage meat
1 onion
1 carrot
½ green pepper
Butter
Salt and pepper
Herbs (sage if pork sausage meat is used) to taste
Tomato puree or ketchup
Egg or milk
Chop the vegetables finely. Mix all the ingredients together (except the tomato puree). Line a pie dish or baking tin with half the pastry and fill with the mixture. Cover with a layer of

tomato puree and close the pie with the remaining pastry. Prick with a fork and brush with beaten egg or milk. Bake at 400°F or Gas No 6 for 45 minutes or until nicely browned.

Marmite whirls

Basic pastry recipe (see page 227)
Marmite
2 oz grated cheese
Roll out the pastry into an oblong. Spread with a thin layer of marmite, sprinkle with grated cheese and roll into a long sausage shape. Cut into thin slices and place on a greased baking sheet. Bake at 425°F or Gas No 7 for about 10 minutes.

Cheese straws

Basic pastry recipe (see page 227)
4–6 oz Cheddar cheese
Salt and pepper
Egg or milk
Roll pastry thinly into an oblong and cover half with grated cheese. Sprinkle with salt and pepper. Fold pastry over and roll out again. Cut into fingers and brush with milk or beaten egg. Bake at 425°F or Gas No 7 for 10–15 minutes or until golden brown.

Tea-time foods

Tea time foods are ones that you must be particularly strong minded about because they all contain sugar and are usually made with white flour. Cakes and biscuits should be kept for special occasions, and the usual food at tea time should be mainly wholemeal bread and plain low-sugar foods. It is difficult to stop having cakes and biscuits completely, because children love them and all their friends have them; but try as hard as you can to reduce these highly refined foods to the absolute minimum.

When baking things for tea you can substitute wholemeal flour for white flour and reduce the sugar in your usual recipes. Adding a small quantity of spices gives more flavour to foods which seem insipid or sour without the usual quantity of sugar. You'll find that a lot of foods have more taste when they are not drowned in sugar and syrups. A teaspoon of sugar is often enough to bring out the flavour of fruit, and it can be added like salt when stewing fruit or sprinkled on in a very small amount before serving.

Extra bran can be added to flour before baking for extra fibre in the proportion of 4 oz bran to 3 lb flour.

Apple cake

8 oz wholemeal flour
2 teaspoons baking powder
½ teaspoon cinnamon or allspice
4 oz butter or margarine
½ lb sweet apples
2 eggs

Topping

1 tablespoon soft brown or demerara sugar
1 teaspoon cinnamon or allspice
1 oz flaked almonds or chopped nuts (optional)
Mix the flour with the baking powder and spice. Rub in the fat and add the coarsely chopped apples and beaten eggs to make a stiff dough. Put the mixture into a tin lined with greaseproof paper.

Mix the ingredients for the topping together and sprinkle over the top of the cake. Bake at 350°F or Gas No 4 for 45–60 minutes. You may like to cover it with greaseproof paper after 30 minutes if it is browning too much.

Tea cakes

2 oz margarine
Generous ¼ pint milk
1 teaspoon sugar
½ oz fresh yeast or 2 teaspoons dried yeast
1 egg
1 lb wholemeal flour
1 teaspoon salt
1 teaspoon mixed spice

2–4 oz sultanas or mixed dried fruit
Melt margarine in a pan, remove from heat and add the milk and sugar. Blend the yeast with the milk mixture and stir in the beaten egg. Leave for 5–10 minutes. Mix the flour, salt, spice and fruit, make a well in the middle and pour in the yeast mixture.

Knead well to a soft dough. Divide into 10 or 12 pieces and shape into rounds. Place on a greased baking sheet and leave to rise in a warm place until double in size (about 30 minutes). Brush with milk and bake in a hot oven (450°F or Gas No 8) for 15–20 minutes. Cool. Serve sliced with butter or toasted and spread with butter while still hot.

Date and walnut loaf

8 oz wholemeal flour
2 teaspoons baking powder
1 level teaspoon bicarbonate of soda
1 teaspoon mixed spice
12 oz chopped dates
1 oz margarine
¼ pint boiling water
1 egg
4 oz chopped walnuts

Mix the flour, baking powder, spice and bicarbonate of soda. Cover the dates and margarine with the boiling water, stir and allow to cool. Mix all the ingredients together and put into a well greased cake or loaf tin. Bake for about 50 minutes at 375°F or Gas No 5.

Banana bread

8 oz wholemeal flour
3 level teaspoons baking powder
Pinch salt
2 oz margarine
1 egg
Grated rind of 1 lemon or rind of 2 oranges
1 teacup mashed banana (about 3 bananas)
Milk

Mix the flour, baking powder and salt and rub in the margarine.

Add the egg, lemon rind and banana pulp and mix thoroughly. You may need to add milk to make the mixture into a sticky consistency. Place in a greased and floured loaf tin and bake for 45 minutes at 375°F or Gas No 5.

Brown scones

8 oz wholemeal flour
Pinch salt
1 level teaspoon bicarbonate of soda
1 level teaspoon cream of tartar
1 oz margarine
Milk to mix
Mix the flour, salt, bicarbonate of soda and cream of tartar and rub in the margarine. Mix to a soft consistency with milk. Knead quickly on a floured board and roll to about ½-inch thickness. Cut into rounds and put on a greased baking sheet. Bake for 15–20 minutes in a hot oven (450°F or Gas No 8). Cool on a wire tray.

These can be served with butter or with jam and cream. They make a special treat when served with mashed banana, strawberries or raspberries and cream.

Rock cakes

8 oz wholemeal flour
2 teaspoons baking powder
1 teaspoon mixed spice
5 oz margarine
1 teaspoon sugar
1 egg
Milk to mix
6 oz dried fruit
2 oz candied peel
Mix the flour, baking powder and mixed spice. Rub in the margarine then add the sugar. Mix in the beaten egg and enough milk to make a stiff consistency. Add the fruit and peel, and place the mixture in small heaps on a greased baking sheet. Bake for 15–20 minutes in the top of a hot oven at 450°F or Gas No 8. Cool on a wire rack.

Nut cookies

2 oz margarine
2 tablespoons sugar
1 egg
2 tablespoons milk
6 oz wholemeal flour
1 teaspoon baking powder
2 oz chopped nuts
2 teaspoons almond essence

Melt the margarine, remove from the heat and stir in the sugar, beaten egg and milk. Mix the flour, baking powder and ginger together and add to the other mixture. Lastly stir in the nuts and almond essence. Roll out thinly and cut into rounds. Bake on a greased baking sheet for 15–20 minutes at 350°F or Gas No 4. Cool on a wire rack.

Fruit cake

6 oz margarine or butter
1 tablespoon sugar (brown or white)
2 eggs
12 oz wholemeal flour
3 level teaspoons baking powder
2 teaspoons mixed spice
1 lb mixed dried fruit
2 oz glace cherries
Milk to mix

Cream the margarine and sugar together, then add the beaten eggs. Mix the flour, baking powder and spice. Mix the cherries and fruit with a little of the flour mixture. Stir the flour into the creamed mixture with enough milk to make a soft consistency. Lastly add the fruit. Put into a greased, floured 8-inch cake tin and bake for 1½–2 hours in the centre of a moderate oven (325–350°F or Gas No 3). For a birthday cake split or flaked almonds can be put on the top of the cake in the initial or age of the child before baking.

Oat cookies

2 oz margarine or butter
2 tablespoons sugar
1 egg
3 oz wholemeal flour
1 teaspoon baking powder
3 oz rolled oats
2 teaspoons almond essence
Milk to mix

Melt the margarine, remove from the heat and stir in the sugar and beaten egg. Add the flour, baking powder, oats and almond essence. Mix to a soft dough with some milk if necessary. Roll out thinly and cut into rounds. Bake on a greased baking sheet for 15–20 minutes at 350°F or Gas No 3. Cool on a wire rack.

Bread making

The best sort of bread is the freshly home-baked loaf and it really is easy to make. The best time to make bread is when you are going to be at home all morning or afternoon but it can be fitted into an evening if you start in good time. I make as many loaves as I can at a time and put several into the freezer compartment of my fridge. It keeps very well if frozen and also keeps in the fridge itself if wrapped in foil or polythene. If you do freeze it don't forget to take the loaf out at least 3 hours before you want to use it.

Special tips for breadmaking

1 Warm the bowl first
2 1 part boiling water to 2 parts cold water produces water of the right temperature
3 There is no need to knead for ages – 5 minutes in the bowl is enough
4 Make the dough fairly sticky
5 Leave the dough to rise in a warm place
6 Make as much as you can and store it in the fridge or freezer
7 Let your husband and the older children have a turn – they will soon offer to make it for you.

Wholemeal bread

3 lb wholemeal flour
1 tablespoon salt
1 tablespoon oil or 1 oz margarine
1½–1¾ pints tepid water
1 oz dried yeast (2 tablespoons) or 2 oz fresh yeast
½ teaspoon sugar

Put the flour into a large bowl, mix in the salt and rub in the margarine or oil. Put the yeast and sugar into a warm bowl, add ½ pint of the warm water, mix well with a fork and leave for 10 minutes. During this time you can grease two 2-lb loaf tins or four 1-lb tins. These should be well greased with margarine or cooking fat.

Make a well in the flour and pour in the yeast mixture. Stir the flour in with a spoon and gradually add the rest of the water. Knead with your hands for about 5 minutes until the dough feels smooth and is of a slightly sticky consistency. I always make a fairly wet dough because it means the loaf is easier to slice and does not fall to bits in the middle. I also knead it in the bowl, not on a floured board, as the books usually say. Leave the dough in a warm place until double in size – about 40–50 minutes – and then knead it again for 5 minutes. Divide into the tins, filling them ⅔-full. Leave for 20 minutes until well risen. Bake in a hot oven (450°F or Gas No 8) for 45 minutes. Cool on a rack.

Wholemeal rolls

These can be made from the same recipe as above and baked at the same temperature for about 35–40 minutes.

Muesli

Muesli has become a very popular breakfast food and forms a very good high-fibre breakfast for the family. It is filling and can easily be made at home. There is a great variety in the shops, but most of them have sugar or honey added and some are much too sweet. There are endless variations which you can try, and you will gradually work out your own recipes, but here are a few suggestions. You can either buy a ready-mixed muesli base and then add nuts, fruit etc to taste, or you can buy the cereal flakes separately and mix them in different proportions. Muesli can be eaten 'raw', or roasted for a short time in the oven. If you roast the mixture add the dried fruit afterwards.

Uncooked muesli 1

1 lb muesli base
2–4 oz chopped nuts
2–4 oz raisins and sultanas
Mix all the ingredients together and store in a tin
Serve with milk.

Variations

1 You can add extra bran either when mixing (2–4 oz to 1 lb muesli base) or when serving individual portions (1 tablespoon bran to 1 portion).
2 Wheatgerm can be added (2–4 oz per 1 lb base)
3 Apple flakes can be added ($\frac{1}{2}$ packet per 1 lb base).

Uncooked muesli 2

$\frac{1}{2}$ lb rolled oat flakes
$\frac{1}{2}$ lb rolled wheat flakes
$\frac{1}{2}$ lb rolled barley flakes
$\frac{1}{4}$ lb millet flakes
$\frac{1}{4}$ lb wheatgerm
6 oz mixed chopped nuts
8 oz sultanas or raisins
Mix the flakes and wheatgerm together and then add nuts and dried fruit. Serve with milk or yoghourt.

Cooked muesli 1

8 oz rolled oats
4 oz wheatgerm
4 oz rolled wheat flakes
3–4 oz coconut (optional)
3 oz bran

2 tablespoons sesame seeds
4 oz chopped walnuts or mixed nuts
1 tablespoon honey (optional)
¼ pint vegetable oil

Combine the oil with the honey and rub into the dry in-gredients. Bake until golden at about 300°F or Gas No 2, stirring every 10 minutes – this takes about ½ hour.

Serve with sliced apple or banana and milk, or mix in 4 oz raisins or sultanas after the mixture has cooled and serve with milk.

Cooked muesli 2

2 oz oil or butter
4 oz rolled oats
2 cups bran flakes
4 oz chopped nuts
4 oz sultanas or raisins

Melt the fat in a heavy pan and add the oats. Cook over a gentle heat until they are brown, stirring from time to time. (or bake in the oven at 300°F or Gas No 2 for 20–30 minutes, stirring occasionally). Let the mixture cool and stir in the bran flakes, nuts and dried fruit. Mix well, cool and store. This is delicious served as a dessert with cream, stewed apple or sliced raw apple or banana.

Section four
Can it really all be true?

Can it really all be true?

Over the last two years that I've been involved with the fibre story, I've been in the closest contact with the doctors and researchers who are in favour of it. But being sceptical by nature I've always tried to throw a spanner into the works whenever possible. This is because as a doctor one is only too well aware that 'miracle cures' are two a penny and that some are even potentially harmful. Many wonder cures of the last decade have been rejected and replaced by new ones – fashions in medicine come and go just as in furnishing or clothes.

Yet for all this one cannot but be impressed by the slow, inexorable grind of progress of a story such as this, which has taken nearly a century to come before the public eye. Fellow doctors and friends threw up their hands in astonishment when I declared my interest, first in making films and then writing a book about 'roughage'. This very attitude has permeated the whole subject ever since Dr Allinson wrote his far-sighted articles in the nineteenth century.

As a doctor, and even more so as a potential patient, I am doubly wary of nutritional fads. Unfortunately, food is an emotive subject and anyone who purports to be thinking afresh about something we all take for granted is all too easily labelled a 'faddist'. It's highly respectable to research the more erudite corners of medicine, but often the bread-and-butter areas are overlooked, because they are just that.

Fibre has only recently become an acceptable medical topic, yet the major specialist journals of the world now have articles on the subject almost every month, and good research is being done at last. But because the subject has been treated, like so many others in nutrition, rather perfunctorily by the medical profession, structured criticism of the fibre story has not really emerged yet. To be quite frank this is mainly because most doctors' knowledge of nutrition is so poor.

This said though, some doctors feel the fibre story is too simple by far, and find it inconceivable that such a simple thing could be happening under our very noses without anyone ever thinking of it before. Others are now prescribing bran and wholemeal bread to a clamouring public – and with gratifying results. But what of the real criticism?

The most important fact to bear in mind is that a large part of the fibre story began with epidemiological evidence gleaned from rural Africa. Studies of populations and their different disease patterns are all very well, but they do not prove anything very much. It's all too easy to pick and choose the data that fit the story you want to put across, and after all not many people (even at a very high medical level) can in fact go off and repeat a study of gallstones in some distant tribe or other. In medicine, just as in any other scientific discipline, one is only as good as one's colleagues and one has to rely on their data, assuming it to be properly collected.

This means that the studies of various nations and their illnesses have to be compared very cautiously. A rarely mentioned fact for instance is that the lining of the bowel of rural Africans is very different from ours in microscopic structure. Is this the cause or the effect of eating lots of fibre? No one knows. Linked to this, may there not be differences at a basic biochemical level in the functioning of our bowels, when compared with those of other peoples? This sort of cellular research hasn't been done in enough communities yet to provide an answer.

Then, is it reasonable to say 'X is common in Scotland' for instance when 'X' is fairly uncommon in some parts of Scotland and very common in others? So many statistics make whole countries, or even continents seem as one – which they're not. Bowel cancer in the USA shows quite a distinct regional distribution, but there doesn't *seem* to be a parallel between geographical variation in fibre consumption and this cancer. Could the actual fall in the number of appendices removed in the USA over the last few years be due to the stricter criteria for removing them, or is it linked to other as yet unknown factors?

There is also good evidence that cancer of the colon may be linked to fat intake – I don't think this possibility can be simply ignored.

Some nutritionists seem to be convinced that taking fibre-rich foods will deplete the body of calcium and iron by binding them to phytic acid, a substance found in cereal fibre. There is evidence both for and against this theory, but on balance I feel that the idea is a red herring. It seems unlikely that anyone eating as much red meat and vegetables as most of us in the West do could in reality go into negative iron balance unless we ate great heaps of fibre – which we couldn't and wouldn't. Still, if you *are* worried by this theory, simply take a little more milk than normal so as to replace the calcium, rather than abandon your High-Fibre Diet.

A lot of the base-line thinking in any medical research is built on animal studies. How justifiable this is, is open to question. Undoubtedly, many body systems of carefully selected animals are so similar to those of man that we can reasonably transfer information learned from one to the other. All too often though we're using animal studies incorrectly. For instance, the diet of laboratory animals often compares in no way either with what the animal would eat if it were in the wild or indeed with our human diet. The food that laboratory animals eat to some extent merely mirrors our impressions of what we think they need. As a result, most laboratory animals used in experiments may well be getting too refined a diet or a diet with some notional 'fibre' added back, which may well not be the same thing as if it had never been removed in the first place. Can we then say that the way their bowels, or indeed their bodies as a whole, respond to other superimposed factors, such as carcinogens, is the same as it would be in the wild?

A good example of this dilemma is to be found in a series of tests carried out on a red food colouring material in America. The colouring matter was found to kill laboratory animals within two weeks, but only if they were eating refined diets. If they were on unrefined food when the colouring matter was fed to them, they lived and even thrived. The scientists responsible for this work highlighted a very important fact – it's no good testing drugs, food additives, cyclamates or whatever on animals and then pronouncing them safe for man unless the diets are comparable. I would add that it's difficult even then to extrapolate from animals to man.

What the fibre story needs is a large prospective study. This would mean taking a large number of people, putting them on high-fibre diets and monitoring all sorts of biochemical and physiological data. They would, of course, have to be age and sex-matched with controls from the same communities so as to rule out local environmental factors. The numbers of people and the sheer volume of investigative procedures needed make this sort of study both expensive and unwieldy, but it's the only real way of proving that we're right about fibre. All other evidence must be second best, though it's the best we've got at present. Unfortunately, some of the diseases we've been discussing have very long 'incubation periods' so our study would have to last for up to forty years – a daunting task. Others of the diseases though, appendicitis and constipation for example, have such a short incubation period that we have already been able to see positive results in present-day studies.

In the meantime there's no doubt in my mind that we *must* proceed on the assumption that high-fibre diets do more good than most other things anyone has come up with for many of the conditions we've been discussing.

Fibre's cheap, as safe as we can say anything is, and it already has a good track record. Just think of the millions of pounds spent every year on foods, patent medicines and drugs of which this can't be said – and it's certainly worth a try. After all . . . '*Heads – you win: tails – you don't lose.*'

Selected bibliography

There are probably well over a thousand scientific papers and articles on the subject of dietary fibre at the time of going to press. Much of this book is the result of long personal contact with those actually doing the research but much of the factual detail can be found in the following books and scientific papers. This is, obviously, only a small selection of the total literature.

Books

Brothwell, D., and Brothwell, P. (1969) *Food in Antiquity*. 162. Thames and Hudson, London.

Burkitt, D. P., and Trowell, H. C., Editors (1975) *Refined Carbohydrate foods and Disease*. Academic Press, London.

Cameron, Allan G. (1971) *Food – Facts and Fallacies*. Faber and Faber Ltd.

Cleave, T. L. (1974) *The Saccharine Disease*. John Wright and Sons Ltd.

Crawford, Michael, and Crawford, Sheilagh (1972) *What We Eat Today*. Neville Spearman.

Curtis-Bennett, Sir Noel (1949) *The Food of the People*. Faber and Faber.

Drummond, J. C., and Wilbraham, A. *The Englishman's Food*. London, 1939.

Fibre in Human Nutrition (1973) Edited A. C. Field. Nutrition Society Symposia Reprint Series No. 5. *Proceedings of the Nutrition Society* 32: 123–167.

Food and Your Health (1974) Selected and abbreviated articles from Consumers' Research Magazine. Edited by Beatrice Trum Hunter. A Pivot Original Health Book.

Hutchinson's Food and the Principles of Nutrition. (1969) 12th Edition. Edward Arnold (Publishers) Ltd, London.

Kent, N. L. (1970) *The Technology of Cereals.* Pergamon Press, Oxford.

McCance, R. A., and Widdowson, E. M. (1956) *Breads White and Brown.* Pitman Medical Publishing Co. Ltd.

McCarrison, R. (1943) *Nutrition and Health.* Faber and Faber Ltd, London.

Painter, N. S. (1975) *Diverticular disease of the colon – A deficiency disease of Western Civilisation.* Heinemann, London.

Trowell, H. C. (1960) *Non-Infective Disease in Africa.* Edward Arnold (Publishers) Ltd, London.

Papers

Adatia, A. K. (1974) *Plant Food for Man.* 1 : 81.

Alexandersen, V. (1967) In *Diseases in Antiquity* (D. Brothwell and A. T. Sandison, eds) 551. Charles C. Thomas, Springfield, Illinois.

Allinson, T. R. (undated) *The Advantage of Whole Meal Bread.* London.

Aries, V., Crowther, J. S., Drasar, B. S., Hill, M. J., and Williams, R. E. O. (1969) *Gut* 10: 334.

Bersohn, I., Walker, A. R. P., and Higginson, J. (1956) 'Coronary Heart Disease and Dietary Fat.' Correspondence. *South African Medical Journal* 30: 411–412.

Brown Bread Versus White (Editorial) (1937) *British Medical Journal* II, 752.

Burch, G. E. (1972) Annotation. *American Heart Journal.* Vol 83, 285–286.

Burkitt, D. P. (1971) 'The Aetiology of Appendicitis.' *British Journal of Surgery* 58: 695–699.

Burkitt, D. P., 'Dietary Fibre and Disease.' *Journal of the American Medical Association* 229: 1068–1074.

Burkitt, D. P. Walker A. R. P., and Painter, N. S. (1972) 'Effect of Dietary Fibre on Stools and Transit-times and its Role in the Causation of Disease.' *Lancet*, December 30: 1408–1441.

Burkitt, D. P. (1972) 'Varicose Veins, Deep Vein Thrombosis and Haemorrhoids: Epidemiology and Suggested Aetiology.' *British Medical Journal* 2: 556–561

Burkitt, D. P., and James, P. A. (1973) 'Low-Residue Diets and Hiatus Hernia.' *Lancet*, July 21: 128–130.

Burkitt, D. P. (1973) 'Cancer and Other Non-infective Diseases of the Bowel. Epidemiology and Possible Causitive Factors.' *Reudic. Gastoenterol.* 5: 33–39.

Cleave, T. L. (1956) 'The Neglect of Natural Principles in Current Medical Practice.' *Journal Royal Naval Medical Service* No. 2 XLII: 55–83.

Davidson, S., and Passmore, R. (1975) *Human Nutrition and Dietetics.* 6th edition. Livingstone, Edinburgh.

Dimoch, E. M. (1937) 'The Prevention of Constipation.' *British Medical Journal* 2: 906–909.

Doll, R. (1969) 'The Geographical Distribution of Cancer.' *British Journal of Cancer* 23: 1–8.

Drasar, B. S., and Hill, M. J. (1972) 'Intestinal Bacteria and Cancer.' *American Journal of Clinical Nutrition* 25: December, 1399–1404.

Eastwood, M. A., *et al.* (1973) 'The Effects of Dietary Supplement of Wheat Bran and Cellulose on Faeces.' *Proceedings of the Nutrition Society* 32: 22A.

Findlay, J. M., Mitchell, W. D., Smith, A. N., Anderson, A J. B., and Eastwood, M. A. (1974) 'Effects of Unprocessed Bran on Colon Function in Normal Subhects and in Diveticular Disease.' *Lancet*, February 2, 146–149.

Greaves, J. P., and Hollingsworth, D. F. (1966) 'Trends in Food Consumption in the United Kingdom.' *Wld Rev. Nutr. Diet* 6: 34–89.

Heaton, K. W. (1973) 'Are We Getting Too Much Out of Food?' *Nutrition*, Lond., XXVII No. 3 170–183.

Heaton, K. W. (1973) 'Food Fibre as an Obstacle in Energy Intake' *Lancet*, December 22, 1418–1421.

Hill, M. J. (1971) 'Bacteria and Aetiology of Cancer of the Large Bowel.' *Lancet* 1: 95–100.

Hinton, J. M., Lennard-Jones, J. E., and Young, A. C. (1969) 'A New Method for Studying Gut Transit Times Using Radioopaque Markers.' *Gut* 10: 842–847.

Keys, A., Anderson, J. T., and Grande, F. (1960) 'Diet Type (Fats Constant) and Blood Lipids in Man.' *Journal of Nutrition* 70: 257–266.

Kritchevsky, D., and Tepper, S. A. (1968) 'Experimental Atherosclerosis in Rabbits Fed Cholesterol Free Diets; Influence of Chow Components.' *Journal of Atherosclerosis Research* 8: 357–369

Latto, C., Wilkinson, R. W., and Gilmore, O. J. A. (1973) 'Diverticular Disease and Varicose Veins.' *Lancet* 1: 1089–1090.

McLaren, D. S. (1972) *Nutrition and its Disorders*. Churchill Livingstone, Edinburgh.

Oliver, M. F., and Stuart-Harris, C. H. (1965) 'Present Position Concerning Prevention of Heart Disease.' *British Medical Journal* 2, 1203.

Painter, N. S. *et al.* (1965) 'Segmentation and the Localisation of Intraluminal Pressures in the Human Colon.' *Gastroenterology* 49: 169–177.

Painter, N. S. (1970) 'Pressures in the Colon Related to Diveticular Disease.' *Proceedings Royal Society of Medicine* 63, Suppl., 144–145.

Painter, N. S. *et al.* (1971) 'Diveticular Disease of the Colon: A Deficiency Disease of Western Civilisation.' *British Medical Journal* 2: 450–454.

Painter, N. S. *et al.* (1972) 'Unprocessed Bran in Treatment of Diverticular Disease of the Colon.' *British Medical Journal* 2: 137–140.

Painter, N. S. (1974) 'Diveticular Disease of the Colon.' *Modern Geriatrics*, January, 8–16.

Poole, D. F. G., and Silverstone, L. M. (1973) In *Hard Tissue Growth, Repair and Remineralisation* – Ciba Foundation Symposium 11 (New Series). 35. ASP (Elsevier), Amsterdam.

Robertson, J. (1972) 'Changes in the Fibre Content of the British Diet.' *Nature* (London) 238: 290–292.

Roche, A. F. (1964) 'Ageing in Man.' *Medical Journal of Australia* 2, 11.

Short, A. R. (1920) 'The Causation of Appendicitis.' *British Journal of Surgery* 8: 171–186.

Trowell, H. (1972) 'Dietary Fibre and Coronary Heart Disease.' *European Journal of Clinical and Biological Research*. Issue 4. Volume 17: 345–349.

Trowell, H. (1972) 'Ischaemic Heart Disease and Dietary Fibre.' *American Journal of Clinical Nutrition* 25: 926–932.

Trowell, H. (1973) 'Dietary Fibre, Ischaemic Heart Disease and Diabetes Mellitus.' *Proc. Nutr. Soc.* 32: 151.

Trowell, H. (1974) 'Diabetes Mellitus Death Rates in England and Wales 1920–70 and Food Supplies.' *Lancet*, October 26, 998.

Trowell, H., Painter, N. S., and Burkitt, D. P. (1974) 'Aspects of the Epidemiology of Diverticular Disease and Ischaemic Heart Disease.' *American Journal of Digestive Diseases*. New Series. Vol 19, No. 9, September, 864–873.

Walker, A. R. P. (1947) 'The Effect of Recent Changes of Food Habits on Bowel Motility.' *South African Medical Journal*, August 23.

Walker, A. R. P. (1955). 'Diet and Atherosclerosis.' Letter to Editor. *Lancet*, March 12, 565–566.

Walker, A. R. P. (1956) 'Some Aspects of Nutritional Research in South Africa.' *Nutrition Review*, Vol 14, No. 11, 321–324.

Walker, A. R. P., and Bersohn, I. (1957) 'Why Atherosclerosis?' *Medicine in South Africa.*

Walker, A. R. P. (1961) 'Crude Fibre, Bowel Motility and Pattern of Diet.' *South African Medical Journal* 35: 114–115.

Walker, A. R. P., and Walker, B. F. (1969) 'Bowel Motility and Colonic Cancer.' *British Medical Journal*. Letter to Editor. 3: 238.

Walker, A. R. P. (1969) 'Bowel Transit Times in Bantu Population.' *British Medical Journal* 3: 238.

Walker, A. R. P. (1969) 'What Can Be Done to Retard Ageing and to Increase Expectation of Life?' *Annals of Life Insurance Medicine* 4: 176–203.

Walker, A. R. P., Walker, B. F., and Richardson, B. D. (1970) 'Bowel Transit Times in Bantu Populations.' *British Medical Journal* 3: 48–49.

Walker, A. R. P. (1971) 'Diet and Cancer of the Colon.' Letter to Editor. *Lancet*, March 20, 593.

Walker, A. R. P. (1971) 'Diet, Bowel Motility, Faeces Composition and Colonic Cancer.' *South African Medical Journal*, 45: 377–379.

Walker, A. R. P. (1971) 'Diet, Bowel Motility, Faeces Composition and Colonic Cancer.' *South African Medical Journal* 45: 377–379.

Walker, A. R. P., Richardson, B. D., Walker, F., and Woolford, A. (1973) 'Appendicitis, Fibre Intake and Bowel Behaviour in Ethnic Groups in South Africa.' *Postgraduate Medical Journal* 49: 243–249.

Walker, A. R. P. (1974) 'Survival Rate at Middle Age in Developing and Western Populations.' *Postgraduate Medical Journal*, January, 50: 29–32.

Index

Adulteration of bread 52, 55–6, 58–60
Alcohol as a food 168–9
Angina pectoris 23, 26, 108
Animals
in food research 243
value of experiments in 106, 243
Appendicitis
and fibre lack 133
causes of 133–4
history 132–3
in African troops 133
in boarding schools 133
in China 133–4
in prisoners 67, 133
what it is 134
Artificial sweeteners 166–7
Atheroma 112, 113, 118, 121

Bacteria
in bowel 46–7, 120, 139, 148, 149, 150, 151
in bowel cancer 150
Bile salts
and cancer 151
and fat digestion 89, 102
Blood
clotting and fibre 119
pressure in primitive people 28
pressure in urban people 28, 29
sugar 89

Body weight
in primitive people 27, 87–8
in urban dwellers 84
Bowel
function of 89
pressures in the 135
pressure measurement 125
Bran
adding bran to food 118, 139, 169–73
how to take it 139, 169–73
laxative effects of 64, 126, 138
on board ship 65, 138
recipes 193 ff
side effects of 170–1
studies of 64, 99
use of 93
what it is 169
Bread
adulteration of 58, 60
brown 49, 55, 158
history of 49, 58–60
making 157
white 55, 58, 76, 92
wholemeal 49, 54, 55, 61, 62, 92, 124, 157, 160

Cancer
and bile salts 151
of the colon 26, 147
Carcinogens in bowel cancer 149, 150

Caries
  and white flour 76–7
  history of 73–4
  how it's caused 74
  in World War 2 77
  on Tristan da Cunha 75–6, 78
  today's problem 73–4
  what it is 74–5
Cellulose 43, 46
Cereals, breakfast 55, 56, 159,
  185
Cholera 24, 25
Cholesterol
  and atheroma 112
  and fibre intake 117, 118
  and gallstones 103, 106
  and heart disease 112, 118, 119
  and obesity 104
  levels in different populations
  114
  production 104
Cigarettes and heart disease 115
Clot(s)
  and fibre 145
  in heart disease 112
  in deep venous thrombosis 144
  prevention with bran 118
Colon
  bran and the 125–7
  cancer 140
  cancer and bacteria 151
  cancer and fats 151
  diverticular disease of the 23,
  46, 126, 127
  function of 46, 89, 125, 148
Constipation
  bran and 65, 130, 138
  causes of 135–40
  definition 137
  treatment of 138, 139

Deep venous thrombosis
  and pulmonary embolus 144

after operations 144
  definition 144
  in Africans 145
  prevention of 146
  treatment of 145
Dentures, children and 74
Deoxycholate
  and gallstone formation 106,
  107
  in colon cancer 149
Diabetes
  history of 95
  in animals 95
  in World War 2 98
  juvenile onset 97, 98, 99
  maturity onset 97, 98
  today 95
Dietary fibre see Fibre
Dietetics, history of 35–7
Digestion
  how it works 90
  of refined foods 89
Diphtheria 24
Diverticular disease of the colon
  23, 46
  and appendicitis 132–5
  and atheroma 121
  and cancer of the colon 147–9
  and heart disease 131
  bran and 67, 125, 139
  in various parts of the world 26,
  122–7
Diverticulitis
  history of 24, 127–9, 131
  frequency 125
  what it is 128

Eating out 183–4
Entertaining 181–3
Epidemics 19, 21
Epidemiology, shortcomings of
  242
Eskimos
  and caries 76

and heart disease 114
Exercise
and heart disease 30, 115
and weight loss 31
Finnish lumberjacks and 116
in primitive communities 29,
92
in urban communities 30
value of 30

Fat
and heart disease 113–15
consumption 37, 149, 167–8
digestion 151
polyunsaturated 114–15
saturated 114, 117, 121
Fibre
and appendicitis 122, 133
and bile salts 151
and bowel cancer 149, 150,
151
and calcium and iron loss 48,
243
and colon cancer 122, 151
and constipation 122, 137, 138,
139
and diarrhoea 139
and digestion 44, 151
and diverticular disease 46, 120,
129, 130, 131
and fat absorption 117, 175
and fatty acids 139
and food absorption 44
and fullness 91
and harmful chemicals 47
and iron exchange 48, 243
and stool bulk 124
and stool weight 46
and tooth decay 81
and transit time 124
and water absorption 45–6, 139,
150
discovery of 41
early research 41, 45

in history 45, 58
rich sources of 49
what it is 41–50
Flour
and dental decay 76
history of 58
white – manufacture 39, 53, 55,
76
wholemeal 55, 63, 195
Food
additives 56
adulteration 52
changes over last century 36,
37, 40, 51
in primitive communities 35,
38, 92
in towns 38
preserving 51
processing 51
transporting 51
Freezers 186–7
Fruit
consumption 49, 54
cooking 220

Gallbladder
anatomy 102
removal of 103
Gallstones
and bacteria 108
formation 103
in animals 102, 106
in developing countries 103,
105
in history 104
in the UK 103
in the USA 103
Glycogen 96, 97
Grain, structure of 39
Growth-rate in children
rural 27
urban 27
Gum disease 73, 75, 79–80

Haemorrhoids
and straining at stool 140, 141
how they're caused 141
theories about 140
treatment for 141
what they are 140
Heart, how it works 111
Heart disease
cause of 110, 111–13
deaths from 22, 109, 110
diverticular disease and 131, 140
epidemic of 109, 110
Eskimos and 114
fats and 113–15
history of 109–10
Indians and 20, 110, 114–15
polyunsaturated fats and 114–
15
rarity in other countries 110,
114
Hemicellulose 43
High Fibre Diet 92, 93, 119, 120,
121, 124, 146, 155, 156, 175–6,
177 ff
Honey 166

Indians, and heart disease 20,
110, 114–15
Insulin 95, 96, 97, 100
Irish, brothers and heart disease
118
Italians, and heart disease 117

Larder, stocking 189
Laxatives
addiction to 136
use of 136–7
Life expectancy
changes in 18, 19
in South African whites 19
in American Jews 19
in Indians 20
through the ages 17–20
today 25

Lignin 43, 139
Low fibre diets 121, 124, 126,
151

Masai, and heart disease in 114
Middle age
and diabetes 97–9
killer diseases of 20–1, 23–9
Milling 53, 58–62

National Flour 65
and diabetes 99
and diverticular disease 131
and other diseases 65

Obesity
and cholesterol 104
and exercise 93
in childhood 86, 100
in history 28, 86–7, 97
in primitive communities 28,
87, 106
in urban communities 87
increased death rate from 29, 85
increased disease in 28, 34, 85

Pancreas, in diabetes 95, 100
Parties 180–1
Pastries 55
Pectin 43, 45
Plague 18
Pollution, and Western diseases
29, 33
Potatoes
and heart disease 118
consumption of 54, 92
Pressure diseases 122, 135, 140,
141, 146
Processing of food 51, 57

Recipes 193 ff
Refined foods, digestion of 89
Rice
brown 49

white 49
Rickets 24, 25
Roller mill
  advantage of 61
  introduction of 60

Scarlet fever 24
Shopping 187–9
Slimming
  and high fibre diet 93
  and potatoes 192
Smallpox 24, 25
Smoking
  and Western diseases 29, 33,
    115
  in rural communities 33
  in urban communities 33
Snacks for children 180–1
Squatting 143
Stonegrinding 60–2
Stools
  early studies of 63–9
  volume 46, 48, 92, 124
Stress
  and heart disease 32, 116
  in rural society 31, 32, 116, 117
  in urban society 24, 31, 32, 116
  the role of in disease 29, 32,
    116, 146
Sugar
  and caries 74–5, 77–9, 179
  consumption 38, 66, 75, 149
  consumption in office workers
    91
  historical consumption 66, 75
  in childhood 86, 100, 179–81
  in cooking 166, 195
  refining 53
  weaning off 160–2, 164–7
  West Indians and 77
Synthetic foods 156, 168

Television, and Western diseases
  29, 32, 33

Toothbrushing 80
Towns
  and life expectancy 20
  changes on moving into 20, 29–
    34
  dangers of living in 25–7
Transit times
  in the West 123
  in Zulus 123
  methods of estimating 122–3
Triglycerides
  and heart disease 118, 119
  and refined diets 119
Tristan da Cunha, and tooth
    decay 75–6, 78
Tuberculosis 24, 25

Varicose veins
  causes of 142
  prevention 143
  surgery for 143
  theories about 142
  treatment for 143
  what they are 142
Vegetables
  consumption 49, 54, 161
  in history 59, 60
  preparation and cooking 161–4
Vegetarians 147, 161–2
Vitamins 36, 178

Western diseases
  history of 24
  rarety 100 years ago 24
Whole foods, cost of 191–2
Wholemeal
  bread, advantages of making
    157
  flour 55, 63, 195
  macaroni and spaghetti 55
World War 2
  fall in incidence of diabetes 98
  fall in incidence of diverticular
    disease 131